FOUNDATION OF EDUCATION:

Application to Nursing Education and Practice

A GUIDE FOR NURSING STUDENTS

ASHLEY A. BANGCOLA, DScN.

Foundation of Education:

Application to Nursing Education and Practice

All rights reserved
Copyright @2021 by
ASHLEY A. BANGCOLA

Published by
Lulu Press Inc.
United States of America

ISBN 978-1-329-81774-6

TABLE OF CONTENTS

Copyright page	....	ii
Table of contents	....	iii
Preface	....	iv
SECTION 1	Perspectives on Teaching and Learning...............	1
Chapter 1	Overview of Education in Health Care.....................	3
Chapter 2	Ethical and Legal Foundations of the Educational Process	11
Chapter 3	Applying Learning Theories to Healthcare Practice	19
SECTION II	Characteristics of the Learner............................	27
Chapter 4	Determinants of Learning	29
Chapter 5:	Developmental Stages of the Learner	41
Chapter 6	Motivation, Compliance, and Health Behaviors of the Learner	51
Chapter 7	Gender, Socioeconomic, and Cultural Attributes of The Learner	63
Chapter 8	Special Populations...	75
SECTION III:	Techniques and Strategies for Teaching and Learning......	
Chapter 9	Behavioral Objectives..	89
Chapter 10	Instructional Methods	105
Chapter 11	: Instructional Materials	115
Chapter 12	Technology in Education	121
Chapter 13	Instructional Settings	129
Chapter 14	Evaluation in Healthcare Education	139
Notes	....	154

PREFACE

This book on Foundation of Education and its Application to Nursing Education and Practice serves as a framework for students to learn about nursing education and provide nursing education to patients, their families, fellow staff nurses, and nursing students.

The book consists of fourteen (14) chapters divided into three units. These chapters would set the foundation for learning about nursing education and apply the same in practice. This chapter is intended to be a primary resource for graduate students for whom the role of an educator is an essential component of practice. It is designed to help them become proficient in educating others, considering the basic foundations of the education process, the needs and characteristics of the learner, and the appropriate instructional techniques and strategies for teaching and learning. These will be discussed in the succeeding pages.

I aim to be your partner in learning more about nursing education. At the end of this course, you are expected to be able to demonstrate the ability to communicate effectively using oral, written, and information technology for professional delivery of nursing care, properly evaluate the health needs of diverse populations for necessary teaching based on nursing knowledge to promote health and prevent illness and injury, and finally, exhibit an ongoing commitment to professional development and value of nursing theories/ethical principles in accordance with ethically responsible, legally accountable, specialist nursing practice.

Although it is difficult to cover everything in this new format, we will do everything humanely possible for you to get the most out of this experience as a student. However, a partnership is both ways. While I will do my best and do everything I can, I would also expect the same from you. With our combined efforts, I am sure that the process of learning will remain unhampered and even enhanced.

Ashley A. Bangcola, DScN

SECTION I
PERSPECTIVES ON TEACHING AND LEARNING

CHAPTER 1
OVERVIEW OF EDUCATION IN HEALTH CARE

Overview:

Chapter 1 examines the history of teaching as part of the professional nurse's duty and provides insight into current health-care trends, which have made patient education a highly visible and needed component of nursing care delivery. This chapter also discussed the general purposes, benefits, and goals of the teaching-learning process, as well as the philosophy of the nurse-patient partnership in teaching and learning, the comparison of the education process to the nursing process, and the identification of teaching and learning barriers. The focus is on the nurse's general role in teaching and learning, regardless of the audience of learners. To carry out their professional tasks efficiently and effectively, nurses must have a fundamental awareness of the principles, practice, and teaching and learning process.

Learning Outcomes:

1. Compare and contrast the education process to the nursing process.
2. Evaluate the reasons why patient and staff education is an important duty for professional nurses.
3. Evaluate the barriers and obstacles to the teaching-learning activities with clients, members of the health team, and others in the work environment

OVERVIEW OF EDUCATION IN HEALTH CARE

I. HISTORICAL FOUNDATIONS FOR THE TEACHING ROLE OF NURSES

Patient education has long been regarded as an important part of the nurse's caregiving responsibilities. The nurse's function as an educator is deeply rooted in the nursing profession's history and evolution.

• Mid-1800s — Nursing was initially recognized as a distinct specialty, and nurses' educational responsibilities were recognized as a vital healthcare endeavour. Nurses focused their teaching efforts not only on patient care, but also on preparing other nurses for professional practice.

Florence Nightingale was the ultimate educator and the founder of modern nursing. She not only founded the first nursing school, but she also taught nurses, physicians, and health officials about the importance of proper conditions in hospitals and homes in order to help patients maintain adequate nutrition, fresh air, exercise, and personal hygiene in order to improve their health.

In the United States, the National League of Nursing Education (NLNE) declared in 1918 that a nurse is primarily a teacher and a health agent, independent of the setting in which practice occurs (DeSantis, & Lipson, 2007).

By 1950, the NLNE had defined teaching skills, developmental and educational psychology, and concepts of the educational process of teaching and learning as areas in the nursing school curriculum that were universal to all (Redman, 1993). The suggestion was that following completion of their basic nursing education, nurses should be prepared to take on the role of a teacher of others.

The American Nurses Association (ANA) has issued declarations on the functions, standards, and qualifications for nursing practice, which include patient instruction.

Furthermore, the International Council of Nurses has long advocated health education as a necessary component of nursing care delivery.

Today, state nurse practice acts (NPAs) universally include teaching within nursing practice responsibilities. Nurses are expected to provide instruction to consumers to assist them to maintain optimal levels of wellness, prevent disease, manage illness, and develop skills to give supportive care to family members.

In addition, the Patient's Bill of Rights, first developed in the 1970s by the American Hospital Association and adopted by hospitals nationwide, has established the rights of patients to receive complete and current information concerning diagnosis, treatment, and prognosis in terms they can reasonably be expected to understand.

II. SOCIAL, ECONOMIC, AND POLITICAL TRENDS AFFECTING HEALTH CARE

- In addition to the professional and legal standards established by many organizations and agencies, there is a growing emphasis on nurses' potential role in teaching activities as a result of social, economic, and political changes affecting the public's health across the country.

- Nurses acknowledge the importance of honing their teaching skills in order to stay up with the demands of patient and staff education. Nurses, on the other hand, are in a unique position to provide health education. They are the healthcare professionals who have the most frequent interaction with patients and their families, are usually the most accessible source of information for consumers, and are the most well-respected of all health professionals.

> **Learning Activity 1:**
>
> Can you think of some of the significant forces in the Philippines affecting nursing practice in particular and the healthcare system in general?

III. PURPOSE, BENEFITS, AND GOALS OF PATIENT AND STAFF EDUCATION

- The purpose of patient education is to increase the competence and confidence of clients for self-management.

- The goal of nurses is to support patients through the transition from being invalids to being independent in care, from being dependent recipients to being involved participants in the care process, and from being passive listeners to active learners.

- The single most important action of nurses as caregivers is to prepare patients and their families for self-care. If clients cannot independently maintain or improve their health status when on their own, we have failed to help them reach their potential.

- The benefits of effective patient education are many. Patient education has demonstrated its potential to:

    1. Increase consumer satisfaction
    2. Improve the quality of life
    3. Ensure continuity of care
    4. Decrease patient anxiety
    5. Effectively reduce the incidence of complications of illness
    6. Promote adherence to healthcare treatment plans
    7. Maximize independence in the performance of activities of daily living
    8. Energize and empower consumers to become actively involved in the planning of their care

IV. **THE EDUCATION PROCESS DEFINED**

The educational process is a systematic, sequential, and well-planned sequence of events that includes two fundamental interdependent operations: teaching and learning. The instructor and the student are two interdependent players in this process, which creates a continuous cycle. They collaborate on teaching and learning activities, resulting in mutually desired behavioral changes. Both the student and the teacher benefit from these adjustments. As a result, teaching and learning should always be a collaborative, participatory activity.

The educational process has long been likened to the nursing process, and for good reason: the steps in both processes are nearly identical. They do, however, have distinct goals and objectives.

Similarities of education process and nursing process

Like the nursing process, the education process consists of the basic elements of assessment, planning, implementation, and evaluation. The nursing process and the education process are logical, scientifically based frameworks for nursing. Both processes provide a rational basis for nursing practice rather than an intuitive one. They are methods for monitoring and judging the overall quality of nursing interventions based on objective data and scientific criteria.

Differences of education process and nursing process

The two are different in that the nursing process focuses on the planning and implementation of care based on the assessment and diagnosis of the physical and psychosocial needs of the patient. In contrast, the education process identifies instructional content and methods based on evaluating and prioritizing the client's learning needs, readiness to learn, and learning styles. The outcomes of the nursing process are achieved when the physical and psychosocial needs of the client are met. The outcomes of the education process are achieved when changes in knowledge, attitudes, and skills occur.

V. **ROLE OF THE NURSE AS EDUCATOR**

A partnership mindset should surely inform the nurse's position as a teacher of patients and families, nursing staff, and students.

The nurse should function as a facilitator, facilitating learning by establishing an environment that encourages people to want to learn and allows them to do so

Transferring responsibility for learning from the nurse to the patient is a more self-care-oriented strategy in patient education. As a result, rather than using a didactic teaching technique, the focus should be on supporting learning (Knowles, 1989).

VI. BARRIERS TO EDUCATION AND OBSTACLES TO LEARNING

Many educators have said that adult learning occurs not by the teacher's initiating and motivating the learning process but rather by removing or reducing obstacles to learning and enhancing the process after it has begun. Unfortunately, numerous barriers confront nurses in carrying out their responsibilities for educating clients, and various obstacles can potentially interfere with learning.

Barriers to Education – are those factors impeding the nurse's ability to deliver educational services.

The following are the key organizational, environmental, educational, and clientele factors that serve as impediments to educating others:

1. Lack of time to teach - is cited by nurses as the greatest barrier to carrying out their role effectively as an educator.
2. Lack of skills – Many nurses and other healthcare personnel are traditionally ill-prepared to teach.
3. The nurse educator's characteristics (i.e., motivation to teach) play an important role in determining the outcome of teaching-learning interaction.
4. Low priority is often assigned to patient and staff education by the administration and supervisory personnel.
5. The lack of space and privacy in the various environmental settings where nurses are expected to teach and learners are expected to learn is not always conducive to teaching. Noise, frequent interferences, treatment schedules, and the like negatively affect concentration and effective interaction.
6. An absence of third-party reimbursement to support patient education programs relegates teaching and learning to less than high-priority status.
7. Concerns about coercion and violation of free choice, based on the belief that patients have a right to choose and cannot be forced to comply, explain why some professionals decide not to invest time and effort in

teaching.

8. The type of documentation system used by healthcare agencies has an effect on the quality and quantity of patient teaching recorded

Obstacles to Learning – are those factors that negatively affect the ability of the learner to attend to and process information.

Some of the key impediments to a learner's capacity to pay attention to and comprehend information are listed below (Glanville, 2000):

1. Acute and chronic sickness stress, anxiety, sensory deficiencies, and inadequate literacy in patients are only a few issues that might reduce learner motivation and obstruct the learning process.
2. A client's active position in health decision-making and involvement in the teaching-learning process might be hampered by the negative impact of the hospital environment, which can result in a loss of control, lack of privacy, and social isolation.
3. A lack of learning time as a result of a patient's fast discharge from treatment might discourage and frustrate the learner, limiting their ability and willingness to learn.
4. The learner's personal traits have a significant impact on the degree to which predefined behavioral outcomes are met. Learning styles, readiness to learn, motivation, and compliance, as well as developmental stage traits and learning styles, are all important elements in the success of educational undertakings.
5. The amount and complexity of behavioral adjustments required can overwhelm learners, preventing them from focusing on and achieving learning objectives and goals.
6. Learning potential is hampered by a lack of assistance and continual positive reinforcement from the nurse and others.
7. Psychological barriers to behavioral change include denial of learning needs, resentment of authority, and a lack of desire to take responsibility (locus of control).

8. The healthcare system's inconveniency, complexity, inaccessibility, fragmentation, and dehumanization frequently lead to frustration and abandonment of the learner's efforts to engage in and comply with the learning goals and objectives.

SUMMARY

Many challenges and opportunities are ahead for nurse educators in delivering health care as this nation moves forward in the twenty-first century. The foremost challenge for nurses is to demonstrate, through research and action, that a definite link exists between education and positive behavioral outcomes of the learner. In this era of cost containment, government regulations, and healthcare reform, the benefits of patient and staff education must be made clear to the public, healthcare employers, healthcare providers, and payers of healthcare benefits. To be effective and efficient, nurses must be willing and able to work collaboratively with other healthcare team members to provide consistently high-quality care to the consumer. The responsibility and accountability of nurses for the delivery of care to the consumer can be accomplished, in part, through education based on solid principles of teaching and learning. The key to effective education for patients, families, and nursing staff is the nurse's understanding of and ongoing commitment to educator role.

REVIEW QUESTIONS

a. How far back in history has teaching been a part of the professional nurse's role?

b. What is the overall outcome the nurse educator wants the learner to achieve due to the teaching-learning process?

c. Why is patient/staff education an important issue today in healthcare delivery?

d. What current socioeconomic trends impacting health care are making it imperative that clients and nursing staff be adequately educated?

e. How does the education process parallel the nursing process?

f. How are the terms *education, teaching,* and *instruction* different from but interdependent with one another?

g. How are *barriers to education* different from *obstacles to learning*?

h. What common factor serves as both a barrier to education as well as an obstacle to learning?

CHAPTER 2
ETHICAL AND LEGAL FOUNDATIONS OF THE EDUCATIONAL PROCESS

Overview

The purpose of this chapter is to provide the ethical and legal foundations that underpin the patient education initiative on the one hand and the rights and responsibilities of the provider on the other hand. This chapter explores the differences between and among ethical, moral, and legal concepts. It explores human rights' ethical and legal foundations and reviews health care's ethical and legal dimensions. Furthermore, it examines the importance of documentation of patient teaching that must be considered in the delivery of patient education in healthcare settings.

Learning Outcomes:

1. Synthesize the ethical and legal dimensions of the healthcare delivery system, including patient education
2. Integrate the different ethico-legal principles and standards as a guiding tool (for future nursing administration) in clinical decision-making as deemed applicable in professional nursing practice

ETHICAL AND LEGAL FOUNDATIONS OF THE EDUCATIONAL PROCESS

I. A Differentiated View of Ethics, Morality, and the Law

The legal system and its rules are founded on ethical and moral ideas that society has accepted as behavioral norms over time and through experience (Lesnick and Anderson, 1962). This relationship explains why the phrases ethical, moral, and legal are frequently used interchangeably but are not necessarily synonymous.

The guiding principles of behavior are referred to as ethics.

The term "ethical" relates to behavior norms or standards.
Although the terms moral and morality are sometimes used interchangeably with the terms ethics and ethical, moral rights and obligations can be distinguished from ethical rights and duties.

The term "moral" refers to an individual's internal value system (the "moral fiber" of their being). Externally, this value system, which is characterized as morality, is manifested through ethical action.

Because ethical principles deal with intangible moral ideals, they cannot be enforced by law and are not laws in and of themselves.
Legal rights and duties, on the other hand, are laws that control behavior or conduct and are enforced under threat of punishment or consequence, such as a fine or imprisonment.
Because of the complex relationship between ethics and the law, terms like informed consent, secrecy, non-malfeasance, and justice can be found in the legal system's lexicon.

To follow this line of thinking, nurses may cite *professional commitment* or *moral obligation* as the reason for educating their clients as one dimension of their role. The legitimacy of this role stems from the nurse practice act in force in the particular state where the nurse resides, is licensed, and is employed. Therefore, the nurse practice act is legally binding and protected by the state's police authority in the interest of protecting the public (Brent, 2001).

II. <u>Application of Ethical And Legal Principles to Patient Education</u>

Six fundamental ethical principles underlying the ethical and legal duties involved in the patient education process are intricately woven throughout the ANA's Code of Ethics for Nurses with Interpretive Statements (2001) and the AHA's Patient's Bill of Rights (1975). Autonomy, truthfulness, confidentiality, non-malfeasance, beneficence, and fairness are the guiding values.

1. Autonomy. The autonomy principle relates to the patient's right to self-determination, which safeguards the patient's ability to make decisions on his or her own. The law mandates that "every individual receiving health care be informed in writing of his or her right under state law to make decisions about his or her health care, including the right to refuse medical and surgical care and the right to initiate advance directives," either at the time of hospital admission or before the initiation of care or treatment in a community health setting.

2. Truthfulness, or veracity, is inextricably tied to informed decision-making and informed consent. In 1994, the famous Cardozo judgment (Schloendorff v. Society of New York Hospitals) established a person's fundamental freedom to make decisions about his or her own body. This decision established a legal foundation for patient education or instruction about invasive medical procedures, including the truth about the dangers and advantages of these procedures (Boyd et al., 1998; Rankin & Stallings, 2001)

3. The ethical fabric of legal judgements including negligence and/or malpractice is non-malfeasance, or the concept of "do no harm."

• Negligence is defined as "behavior that falls below the legal threshold for protecting others from an undue risk of harm" (Brent, 2001 p. 54).

• Professional negligence refers to actions taken by professionals (such as nurses, physicians, dentists, and lawyers) that fall short of a professional standard of care (Brent, 2001 p. 55).

> As clarified by Lesnick and Anderson in 1962, Brent (2001) reiterates that for negligence to exist, there must be a duty between the injured party and the person whose actions (or nonactions) caused the injury. A breach of that duty must have occurred, the violation of duty must have

13

been the immediate cause of the injury, and the injured party must have experienced damages from the injury.

- *Malpractice* refers to a limited class of negligent activities committed within the scope of performance by those pursuing a particular profession involving highly skilled and technical services (Lesnick & Anderson, 1962 p.234).

  Thus malpractice is limited in scope to those whose life work requires special education and training dictated by specific educational standards. In contrast, negligence embraces all improper and wrongful conduct by anyone arising out of any activity.

1. **Confidentiality** refers to privileged information or a social contract or covenant in legal terms. The nurse-patient relationship is considered to be privileged in most states. As a consequence, the nurse may not disclose information acquired in a professional capacity from a patient without the consent of the patient "unless the patient has been the victim or subject of a crime, the commission of which is the subject of legal proceeding in which the nurse is a witness" (Lesnik & Anderson, 1962, p. 48).

   This discussion of confidentiality gives rise to the need to distinguish between the concepts of what is *private*, what is *privileged*, and what is *confidential*.

The diagnosis of acquired immune deficiency syndrome (AIDS) provides an excellent opportunity to clarify these issues. Despite the fact that AIDS is contagious, a person diagnosed with the disease is protected by federal and state legislation. AIDS is classified as private information in this situation. It is not necessary to inform others about it at work, at home, or in other social settings. This information is deemed extremely personal under federal law (and in some states), and its privacy is viewed as a fundamental right of the individual. In essence, the Constitution protects this right (Brent, 2001). AIDS is sometimes regarded as privileged information. The patient is the exclusive owner of this information, and it can only be shared with him or her at his or her discretion. This information can only be shared between the nurse and the client unless the client gives permission for it to be shared with other health professionals (Brent, 2001). The diagnosis of AIDS is likewise kept private under the law. As a result, anyone who is not involved in a client's care has no right to confidential or privileged information about the client's health (Brent, 2001).

2. Beneficence. The notion of beneficence (doing good) is legalized by adherence to job descriptions' important responsibilities and obligations, the healthcare facility's rules, procedures, and protocols, and professional nursing organizations' norms and codes of ethical behavior. The nurse's commitment to acting in the best interests of the patient is demonstrated by adherence to these numerous professional performance requirements and principles, including proper and current patient education. Under the prospect of litigation, such behavior focuses patient welfare and deemphasizes the provision of excellent care.

3. Justice refers to the allocation of commodities and services in a fair and equitable manner. The legal system is referred to as the "Justice System." The objective of law is on societal protection; the focus of health legislation is on consumer protection. In most places, the Patient's Bill of Rights is legally enforceable. This means that if a nurse or other health professional discriminates in the provision of care, they may face penalties or legal action. The client has a right to proper teaching regarding the risks and advantages of intrusive medical procedures, regardless of their age, gender, physical impairment, sexual orientation, or race. He or she also has a right to proper education about self-care activities, such as home dialysis, which are outside of most people's typical daily routines.

III. **Legality of Patient Education and Information**

The Patient's Bill of Rights, established by the American Hospital Association in 1975, spells out the patient's right to proper information about his or her physical condition, prescriptions, hazards, and access to information about alternative therapies. Many countries have included these rights into their health legislation, making them legal and enforceable. The rights of patients to education and instruction are likewise governed by accrediting bodies' requirements.

Documentation (fourth)

Patient teaching has been characterized as the "probably the most undocumented skilled service because nurses do not realize the scope and complexity of the instruction they conduct," according to Casey (1995). (p. 257).

The lack of documentation also implies a failure to follow the requirements of the nurse practice legislation in question. Because patient records might be subpoenaed for court evidence, this sloppiness is undesirable. Appropriate documentation can be the deciding factor in a lawsuit's outcome. In other words, if the instruction isn't written down, it didn't happen.

V. Patient Education's Future Directions

Patient education has long been a priority for hospitals and other healthcare organizations. This process, as we all know, frequently takes place at the bedside, in clinic waiting rooms, or in groups on hospital grounds. Some components of this well-known educational process will almost probably be maintained because it is beneficial to the patient's release planning and, in the long run, is cost-effective for the institution. Patient education will take on new dimensions, according to many experts (Abruzzese, 1992; Anderson, 1990). The following dimensions may be included, but are not limited to:

1. The majority of training will take place in the ambulatory care setting.

2. Computer-based training in hospitals, mobile care settings, doctors' offices, and homes will become more common.

3. There will be a rise in the use of interactive video programs.

4. The number of wellness screening programs will rise.

5. With varied educational offers, the emphasis on illness prevention and health promotion, such as nutrition, diet, and exercise, will expand.

6. The number of inter-organizational collaborations in the patient education enterprise will grow.

7. As cost-benefit ratios reveal the cost-effectiveness of consumer education, third-party reimbursement will rise.

SUMMARY: Human rights include ethical and legal elements that require patient education, especially when it comes to questions of self-determination and informed consent. These rights are enforced at the local level through state rules and performance requirements issued by certifying authorities and professional associations. The definition of nursing practice established by the prevailing nurse practice act in the state where the nurse is licensed and employed legitimizes the nurse's position as an educator. In this regard, regardless of the patient's culture, colour, or ethnicity, the nurse has a legal obligation to give patient education. As a result, all clients have a legal right to health education that is tailored to their specific physical and mental needs. Education programs should also be created to align with corporate goals while also satisfying the needs of patients to be informed, self-directed, and in control of their health, according to justice.

REVIEW QUESTIONS

1. How do the terms *ethical, moral, legal* differ from one another?
2. Concerning ethical, moral, and legal obligations, how does the American Hospital Association's *Patient's Bill of Rights* compare to the American Nurses' Association's *Code of Ethics for Nurses with Interpretive Statements?*
3. What are the six ethical principles that dictate the actions of healthcare providers in delivering services to clients?
4. Why are nurse practice acts so important to nurses in carrying out their roles and responsibilities to the public?
5. What is the difference between the terms *negligence* and *malpractice*?
6. When was informed consent established as a basic tenet of ethics, and what is the nurse's role in situations involving informed consent?
7. Why is documentation of professional nursing duties, particularly patient education, so important in the provision of care by nurses?

CHAPTER 3
APPLYING LEARNING THEORIES TO HEALTHCARE PRACTICE

Overview:

This chapter reviews the principal learning theories and is organized as follows: First, the basic principles of learning advocated by a behaviorist, cognitive, social learning, psycho-dynamic, and humanistic theories are summarized and illustrated with examples from health care. Next, these theories are compared about (1) their fundamental procedures for changing behavior, (2) the assumptions made about the learner, (3) the role of the educator in encouraging learning, (4) sources of motivation, and (5) ways in which learning is transferred to new situations and problems. Finally, some common features of learning are identified concerning the issues raised earlier about ways that learning occurs, the kinds of experiences that promote the learning process, and ways to ensure that learning is relatively permanent.

Learning Outcomes:
1. Define the principal constructs of each learning theory.
2. Give an example applying each theory to changing the attitudes and behaviors of learners in a specific situation.
3. Outline alternative strategies for learning in a given situation using at least two different learning theories.

APPLYING LEARNING THEORIES TO HEALTHCARE PRACTICE

Learning is a relatively permanent change in mental processing, emotional functioning, and/or behavior due to experience. It is the lifelong, dynamic process by which individuals acquire new knowledge or skills and alter their thoughts, feelings, attitudes, and actions. Despite the significance of learning to human development, it has long been debated how learning occurs, what kinds of experiences facilitate or hinder the learning process, and what ensures that learning becomes relatively permanent.

LEARNING THEORIES

A learning theory is a set of integrated constructs and concepts that describe, explain, or predict how people learn. Rather than providing a single theory of learning, educational psychology offers a variety of theories and viewpoints on how people learn and why they change (Bigge & Shermis, 1992; Hilgard & Bower, 1966; Hill, 1990).

1. **Behaviorist Learning Theory** - considers learning to be a product of stimulus conditions (S) and subsequent reactions (R)—also known as the S-R model of learning.

Behaviorists propose either modifying the stimulus conditions in the environment or changing what happens after a reaction occurs to change people's attitudes and responses.

Respondent conditioning (also known as classical or Pavlovian conditioning) highlights the significance of stimulus conditions and connections created during the learning process (Klein & Mowrer, 1989). A neutral stimulus (NS)—a stimulus with no particular value or meaning to the learner—is matched with a naturally occurring unconditioned or unlearned stimulus (UCS) and the unconditioned response (UCR) in this basic model of learning (UCR). After a few such pairings, the neutral stimulus alone evokes the same response as the unconditioned stimulus. Learning occurs when the freshly conditioned stimulus (CS) becomes connected with the conditioned response (CR). It often happens without thought or awareness (CR).

Consider the health-care industry. Someone with little hospital experience (NS) might pay a visit to a sick relative. The visitor may detect foul odors (UCS) and feel nauseated and light-headed when in the relative's room (UCR). Hospitals (now the CS) may become associated with feeling uncomfortable and sick (CR) after this initial visit and subsequent trips, especially if the visitor detects aromas similar to those detected during the first experience. The importance of the "environment" and staff morale in health care is highlighted by respondent conditioning. Patients and visitors establish these associations as a result of their hospital experiences, sometimes without thinking or thought, laying the groundwork for long-term views about medicine, healthcare facilities, and health professionals.

Operant conditioning is concerned with the behavior of the organism and the reinforcement that follows the response (Alberto & Troutman, 1990). A reinforcer is a stimulus or event given after a response that increases the likelihood that the reaction will be repeated. Behaviors can be increased or lessened when certain responses are reinforced on a regular basis.

Families of chronic back pain patients, for example, have been taught to pay close attention to their loved ones when they complain and behave in helpless, dependent ways, but to pay close attention when they try to function independently, express a positive attitude, and live as normal a life as possible.

2. Cognitive Learning Theory - emphasizes the significance of what happens "within" the learner (Brien & Eastmond, 1994).

Cognition is the key of learning and change (perception, thought, memory, and ways of processing and structuring information).

Individuals must adapt their cognitions to learn, according to this viewpoint. Perceiving information, evaluating it based on prior knowledge, and then reorganizing the information into new insights or understanding are all part of learning (Tatman & Gilgen, 1999).

3. **According to Social Learning Theory,** learning is generally a social process in which other people, particularly "important ones," provide compelling examples or role models for thinking, feeling, and doing.

According to early social learning theory, a lot of learning happens through observation—observing other people and figuring out what they do.

4. **Psychodynamic Learning Theory** – emphasizes the importance of conscious and unconscious forces in guiding behavior, personality conflicts, and the long-term effects of childhood experiences; the psychodynamic perspective emphasizes the importance of conscious and unconscious forces in guiding behavior, personality conflicts, and the long-term effects of childhood experiences.
One of the theory's fundamental tenets is that conduct can be conscious or unconscious—that is, people might be aware of their motivations and why they feel, think, and act the way they do or not.

The id, according to psychodynamic theory, is the most primal source of motivation. Dry, uninteresting lectures delivered by health professionals who go through the motions of the presentation without any enthusiasm or emotion inspire few people to listen or obey the advice, according to Freud. It acts on the pleasure principle—to seek pleasure and avoid pain.

5. **Humanistic Learning Theory** - The humanistic learning theory is based on the concept that each individual is unique and that everyone wants to grow in a positive way.

The humanistic approach, like psychodynamic theory, is primarily a motivational theory. Motivation is derived from each person's needs, subjective thoughts about oneself, and desire to progress, according to a humanistic approach.

➢ Curiosity, a positive self-concept, and open environments where individuals appreciate individuality and support freedom of choice aid learning transfer. Under such circumstances, the transfer is likely to be widespread, resulting in increased flexibility and creativity.

> **Learning Activity 2:**
>
> In a table, provide a comparative summary of the five learning theories outlined in this chapter in terms of each theory's (1) learning procedures; (2) assumptions about the learner; (3) educator's task; (4) sources of motivation; and (5) transfer of learning.
>
> Which of these five theories "best" describes or explains learning—which theory, in other words, would be the most helpful to health professionals interested in increasing knowledge or changing the behavior of patients, staff, or themselves?

I. COMMON PRINCIPLES OF LEARNING

Learning, according to the ideas described in this chapter, is a more complicated process than any single theory suggests. By integrating the learning theories and finding their common principles, the difficulties stated at the beginning of the chapter can be addressed.

A. How Does Learning Take Place?

Individuals learn through interacting with their surroundings and combining new information or experiences with what they already know or have learned.

The society and culture, the structure or pattern of stimuli, the effectiveness of role models and reinforcements, feedback for successful and erroneous answers, and opportunities to process and apply learning to new situations are all factors in the environment that affect learning.

Individuals have a great deal of control over their learning, which is influenced by their developmental stage, history (habits, cultural conditioning, socialization, childhood experiences, and conflicts), cognitive style, self-regulation dynamics, conscious and unconscious motivations, personality (stage, conflicts, self-concept), and emotions.

Taking in information is often preferred by students (visual, motor, auditory, or symbolic). Some people learn best on their own, while others gain from professional instruction, social engagement, and cooperative learning.

Motivation has a significant impact on whether or not learning occurs.

B. What Kinds of Experiences Help or Hurt the Learning Process?

Educators must know (the subject to be learnt, the learner, the social context, and educational psychology) and be competent in order to be effective (be imaginative, flexible, and able to employ teaching methods; display solid communication skills; and can motivate others).

Lack of clarity and meaning in what is to be learned, neglect or harsh punishment, fear, negative or ineffective role models, and rewards for unhealthy behavior, confusing reinforcement, and inappropriate materials for the individual's ability, readiness to learn, or stage of life-cycle development are all examples of learning impediments.

Furthermore, people who have had negative socialization experiences, are deprived of stimulating circumstances, and lack goals and realistic expectations for themselves are unlikely to want to learn.

C. What Factors Contribute to Learning Being Relatively Permanent?

First, by arranging the learning experience, making it relevant and delightful, and pacing the presentation in accordance with the learner's ability to assimilate information, the possibility of learning is increased.

Second, putting new knowledge or skills to the test (mentally and physically) in a variety of situations improves learning.

The final point to consider is reinforcement. Although reinforcement may or may not be required, some theories say that it is beneficial since it signals to the individual that learning has taken place (Hill, 1990).

A fourth factor to assess is whether learning is transferable outside of the initial educational setting. Learning cannot be presumed to be relatively long-lasting or permanent; it must be tested and evaluated immediately following the learning experience, as well as through follow-up measurements. The comments from the evaluation can then be used to improve and refresh learning experiences.

SUMMARY

This chapter highlights how difficult learning may be. The different theories, learning concepts, and cautions involved with using the various methodologies may overwhelm readers. Nonetheless, each theory, like the blind man exploring the elephant, focuses on a key aspect that influences the whole learning process. The ideas, when combined, offer a plethora of complimentary techniques and alternate possibilities. Of course, there is no one-size-fits-all method to learning, but all theories point to the importance of being aware of each learner's individual features and motivations. It is unrealistic to expect health care providers and educators to be experts in the learning process. Perhaps more importantly, they can discern what information is required, where to obtain it, and how to assist others in directly benefiting from a learning experience.

REVIEW QUESTIONS

1. What are the five (5) major learning theories discussed in this chapter?
2. What are the principal constructs of each of the five learning theories?
3. According to the Operant Conditioning Model, what are three (3) techniques to increase the probability of a response, and what are two (2) techniques to decrease or extinguish the likelihood of a response?
4. Each cognitive perspective discussed in the chapter focuses on a particular feature of cognition in the learning process. What contribution does each of the following perspectives help us understand the cognitive learning process: gestalt, information processing, developmental, social constructivist, and social cognition? Write one sentence describing the contribution of each perspective.
5. How do the major learning theories compare to one another about their

similarities and differences? Give examples of the ways that various learning theories are similar and how they differ.

6. How does motivation serve as the critical influence on whether learning occurs or not?

7. What kinds of experiences facilitate learning, and what sorts of experiences hinder the learning process?

8. What factors help ensure that learning becomes relatively permanent? Give examples.

SECTION II
CHARACTERISTICS OF THE LEARNER

CHAPTER 4
DETERMINANTS OF LEARNING

Overview:

In various settings, nurses are responsible for educating patients, families, nursing staff, other healthcare staff, and nursing students. Several factors have made using principles of learning particularly challenging for the nurse educator to meet learners' needs for information. To meet these challenges, the nurse educator must know what determines how well a person learns. This chapter will address the determinants of learning concerning the patient teaching and staff education component of nursing practice.

Learning Outcomes

After completing this chapter, the student will be able to:

1. State the nurse educator's role in the learning process.
2. Describe the steps involved in the assessment of learning needs.
3. Explain methods that can be used to assess learner needs.
4. Describe what is meant by learning styles
5. Discriminate between the major learning styles identified

DETERMINANTS OF LEARNING

Nurses are responsible for the education of patients, families, staff, and students in a variety of settings. The nurse educator's responsibility in satisfying the information demands of these distinct categories of learners is particularly difficult due to a number of issues. Furthermore, students are enrolling in nursing schools at an older age, bringing with them a variety of life experiences as well as the obligations of working and having a family while continuing their education. Nurse educators must regularly review the determinants of learning for the various audiences of learners they educate as a result of these and other shifting healthcare trends and population demographics. To tackle these challenges, the nurse educator must understand the numerous aspects that influence a person's ability to learn. This chapter focuses on these three learning factors and how they affect the delivery of effective and efficient patient, student, and staff education. The three factors of learning (McCoy, & Haggard, 1989) are examined while assessing the learner:

1. Learning needs (*what* the learner needs to learn)
2. Readiness to learn (*when* the learner is receptive to learning)
3. Learning style (*how* the learner best learns)

I. **THE EDUCATOR'S ROLE IN LEARNING**

One of the most important interventions a nurse can make is to educate others. To do so effectively, the nurse must first determine what knowledge learners require, as well as their readiness to learn and learning styles. The student is the most important individual in the educational process, not the teacher. When educators work as facilitators, they can help students become more aware of what they need to know, why knowledge is vital, and how to actively participate in learning (Beers, 2003). (2005). An evaluation of the three learning determinants allows the educator to identify material and deliver it in a variety of ways, something a learner cannot do on their own. Learners can experience major parts and wholes by manipulating the environment, allowing them to attain their full potential. By accomplishing the following, the educator plays a critical part in the learning process:

• Identifying issues or deficiencies

• Providing crucial information and presenting it in a unique and relevant manner.

- Identifying the progress that has been made

- Providing input and ensuring that it is followed up on

- Improving learning through reinforcing new knowledge, skills, and attitudes

- Assessing students' abilities

During the learning process, the educator is critical in providing support, encouragement, and guidance. Without the guidance of an educator, students can make decisions on their own, but these decisions may be limited or incorrect. For example, the nurse helps family members make required modifications in the home setting, such as reducing distractions by having them turn off the television to create a peaceful environment favorable to learning. Based on the student's specific learning needs, readiness to learn, and learning style, the educator supports in developing optimal learning approaches and activities that both support and challenge the learner.

ASSESSMENT OF THE LEARNER

Assessment of learners' needs, readiness, and learning styles is the first and most important step in instructional design, but it is also the most likely to be neglected. Frequently, the nurse dives into teaching before addressing all of the determinants of learning. It is not unusual for patients with the same condition to be taught with the same materials in the same way (McCoy, & Haggard, 1989). The result is that information given to the patient is neither individualized nor based on an adequate educational assessment.

Evidence suggests, however, that individualizing teaching based on prior assessment improves patient outcomes (Corbett, 2003) and satisfaction (Bakas et al., 2009).

Nurses are taught that an assessment should precede any nursing intervention. Few would deny that this is the correct approach, no matter whether planning for giving direct physical care, meeting the psychosocial needs of a patient, or teaching someone to be independent in self-care or the delivery of care.

The nurse in the educator role must become more acquainted and comfortable with all the elements of instructional design, particularly with the assessment phase, because it serves as the foundation for the rest of the educational process.

Assessment of the learner includes attending to the three determinants of learning:

1. Learning needs—what the learner needs and wants to learn
2. Readiness to learn—when the learner is receptive to learning
3. Learning style—how the learner best learns

II. **ASSESSING LEARNING NEEDS**

Learning needs are described as knowledge gaps that exist between a desired and actual level of performance (Healthcare Education Association, 1985). A learning need, in other terms, is a discrepancy between what someone knows and what they need or desire to know. Such discrepancies might occur due to a lack of knowledge, attitude, or expertise. Nurse educators must first assess learning requirements in order to build an instructional plan to address any inadequacies in the cognitive, emotional, or psychomotor domains, which are the three determinants of learning. Once the educator has figured out what needs to be taught, he can figure out when and how the best learning may take place. It is the educator's job to figure out what exactly needs to be learnt and how to communicate the knowledge in a way that the learner will grasp. The steps in determining your learning needs are as follows:

1. Determine who the learner is. Who is the intended audience? Is there a single need if the audience is one person, or do many conditions need to be met? Is there more than one person who is learning? If so, are their requirements similar or dissimilar? The creation of formal and informal education programs for patients and their families, nursing staff, or students must be founded on precise learner identification. For example, an educator may consider that all parents of asthmatic children should attend a formal class on home dangers. This impression may be based on the educator's interactions with a small number of patients, and it may not apply to all families. Similarly, because of an isolated event with one staff member failing to follow established infection control protocols effectively, the management of a healthcare institution may seek an in-service session on infection control documentation for all personnel.

2. Select the appropriate setting. Establishing a trusting environment allows students to feel safe sharing personal information, believe their concerns are heard and valued, and feel appreciated. It is well acknowledged that maintaining privacy and confidentiality is critical to developing a trusting connection.

3. Gather information on the learner. Once the learner has been determined, the educator can assess the population's specific needs by looking into common health concerns or subjects of interest to that group. Following that, depending on the analysis of needs, a literature search can assist the educator in determining the type and extent of information to be included in teaching sessions, as well as educational strategies for teaching a specific demographic.

4. Gather information from the learner. Learners are typically the most essential source of data for self-assessment needs. Allow patients and/or family members to choose what is essential to them, what their perceived requirements are, what types of social support systems are accessible, and what kind of help these supports may provide. If the audience for your instruction is made up of staff or students, ask them about the areas of practice where they feel they need new or more information. Learners are more motivated to learn when they are actively involved in defining their challenges and needs. They are invested in creating a curriculum that is suited to their specific needs. Also, because, as previously said, the educator may not always see the same learning needs as the learner, the learner must be included as a source of information.

5. Include members of the healthcare team in the process. As a result of their frequent interactions with both consumers and caregivers, other health professionals are likely to have insight into patient or family needs, as well as the educational needs of nursing staff or students. Nurses are not these people's only teachers, therefore they must remember to collaborate with other members of the healthcare team to get a more complete picture of their learning requirements. This is especially significant because assessment time is frequently restricted.

Prioritize your requirements. A list of recognized needs can quickly grow long and appear impossible to meet. Maslow's (1970) hierarchy of human needs might assist educators in prioritizing such that the learner's basic needs are met first and foremost before moving on to higher demands. Learning about a low-sodium diet, for example, is impossible if a patient is suffering from basic physiological circumstances like pain and discomfort; these latter demands must be met before any other higher-order learning can take place. When a nurse educator is presented with numerous learning demands in various areas, it can be challenging to set learning priorities. Setting realistic and achievable learning goals is easier when the identified needs are prioritized. It's critical to choose which topics to address, and nurse educators must do so carefully. To promote maximum learning, educators should prioritize learning demands based on the following criteria (Healthcare Education Association, 1985, p. 23):

a. Required: Survival skills or situations in which the learner's life or safety are in jeopardy. This category's learning requirements must be met right away. A patient who has just had a heart attack, for example, should be aware of the signs and symptoms and seek prompt medical attention. A hospital nurse must learn how to do cardiac resuscitation and proper isolation techniques for self-protection.

b. Desirable: Needs that aren't life-critical but are related to well-being or the general ability to deliver high-quality care in situations needing institutional process adjustments. Patients with cardiovascular illness, for example, must be aware of the impact of a high-fat diet on their condition. When hospital management decides to focus more on the appropriateness of patient education materials in relation to the patient populations serviced, nurses should update their knowledge by attending an in-service program.

c. Possible: Needs for information that is useful but not essential or required, or situations when the learning requirement is unrelated to daily activities. For example, because this knowledge is unrelated to the patient's daily activities, the newly diagnosed patient with diabetes mellitus is unlikely to need to know about self-care concerns that arise when flying across time zones or staying in a foreign country.

7. **Determine the educational resources that are available.** Even if the educator recognizes a need, it may be futile to proceed with interventions if the necessary educational resources are unavailable, unrealistic to get, or do not meet the learner's needs. In this scenario, it could be best to concentrate on other needs that have been recognized. A patient with asthma, for example, must learn how to utilize an inhaler and a peak-flow meter. The nurse educator may decide that the best way for this patient to learn is for the nurse to show the use of the inhaler and peak-flow meter first, then enable the patient to do a return demonstration. Assume that the appropriate demonstration/return demonstration equipment is not accessible at that time. In that scenario, it could be best for the nurse educator to inform the patient about the signs and symptoms of poor air exchange rather than canceling the appointment. Following that, the educator would get to work on acquiring the appropriate equipment for future meetings.

8. **Evaluate the organization's needs.** This assessment generates data that represents the organization's climate. What is the philosophy, mission, strategic plan, and goals of the organization? The educator should be aware with the various employee categories' performance standards, as well as job descriptions and hospital, professional, and agency laws. If the organization is focused on health promotion rather than trauma care, for example, the educational focus or emphasis will most likely define the learning needs of both consumers and staff.

9. **Take time management into consideration.** Because time limits are a major stumbling block in the assessment process, Rankin and Stallings (2005) recommend that the instructor emphasize the following key principles about time management:

If the educator wants learners to take charge and become actively involved in the learning process, they must be provided time to express their perceptions of their learning requirements.

b. Learners should be asked what they want to study first because this calms their nerves and allows them to move on to more important material.

c. Assessment can take place at any time and in any place when the educator has official or informal contact with students. The collecting of data does not have to be limited to a predetermined schedule.

d. Giving a patient advance warning that the educator wants to spend time discussing difficulties or needs allows the person to organize his or her thoughts and feelings.

f. During planned assessment interviews, minimizing interruptions and distractions enhances productivity. As a result, the educator may be able to complete in 15 minutes what might usually take an hour under less controlled, more frequently interrupted conditions.

III. **READINESS TO LEARN**

Following the identification of learning needs, the educator must assess the learner's readiness to receive information. When a student shows an interest in learning the information needed to maintain optimal health or improve their professional skills, they are said to be ready to learn. Educators have often observed that when a patient or a member of the staff asks a question, the time is ideal for learning. When a student is ready to learn, he or she is receptive, willing, and able to participate in the process. It is the educator's role to determine when patients or staff are ready to learn, what they need or desire to learn, and how to customize the curriculum to meet the needs of each learner through evaluation. To assess learning readiness, the educator must first understand what needs to be taught, then collect and validate that information using the same methods used to assess learning needs previously, such as making observations, conducting interviews, gathering information from the learner as well as other healthcare team members, and reviewing documentation. These chores must be completed by the educator prior to the start of actual learning. No matter how vital the knowledge is or how much the educator believes the student requires it, if the learner is not ready, the information will not be absorbed. Four types of preparation to learn - (PEEK: physical readiness, emotional readiness, experience readiness, and knowledge readiness) (PEEK: physical readiness, emotional readiness, experiential readiness, and knowledge readiness). These four forms of learning readiness can either be a hindrance or a benefit to learning.

1. Physical Readiness - The educator must evaluate five primary components of physical readiness: ability measures, task complexity, environmental influences, health status, and gender, all of which influence the degree or extent to which learning occurs.

2. Emotional Readiness - To learn, students must be emotionally prepared. Emotional readiness, like physical readiness, involves a number of aspects that must be evaluated. Anxiety level, support system, motivation, risk-taking behavior, state of mind, and developmental stage are all elements to consider.

3. Experiential readiness refers to the learner's prior learning experiences. Before beginning to teach, the educator should analyze if earlier learning experiences have helped students overcome problems or complete new tasks in a favorable or negative way. Someone who has had unpleasant learning experiences is unlikely to be motivated or willing to take a chance on changing or learning new behaviors.

4. The learner's present knowledge base, level of learning capability, and preferred learning style are all factors in knowledge readiness. To identify readiness to learn, these components must be examined, and teaching should be prepared accordingly.

IV. **LEARNING STYLES AND INSTRUMENTS**

Learning style refers to the ways individuals process information (Guild & Garger, 1998). Each learner is unique and complex, with a distinct learning style preference that distinguishes one learner from another.

The learning style models are based on the premise that certain characteristics of style are biological in origin, whereas others are sociologically developed as a result of environmental influences. Recognizing that people have different approaches to learning helps the nurse educator to understand the various educational interests and needs of diverse populations.

Six Learning Style Principles

1. Both the style by which the teacher prefers to teach and the style by which the student prefers to learn can be identified.
2. Teachers need to guard against over-teaching by their own preferred learning styles.
3. Teachers are most helpful when they assist students in identifying and learning through their own style preferences.
4. Students should have the opportunity to learn through their preferred style.
5. Students should be encouraged to diversify their style preferences.
6. Teachers can develop specific learning activities that reinforce each modality or style.

Learning Style Instruments

a. Right-Brain/Left-Brain and Whole-Brain Thinking
b. Field-Independent/Field-Dependent Embedded Figures Test
c. Dunn and Dunn Learning Style Inventory
d. Kolb's Learning Style Inventory
e. Gregorc Style Delineator
f. 4MAT System
g. Gardner's Seven Types of Intelligence

> **Learning Activity 3**
>
> Compare and contrast the different learning style instruments
>
> Which is the most reliable and valid method to determine someone's learning style? What does each of the eight learning style instruments measure?

SUMMARY

This chapter stressed the importance of the assessment phase of learning because the educator must be aware of and know how to determine learning needs, the learner's readiness to learn, and the learner's learning style before planning for any educational encounter. Learning is a complex concept that is not directly seen but can be inferred from permanent changes in the learner's behavior. Learning takes place in all three of the cognitive, psychomotor, and affective domains. Behavioral objectives for these three domains should not be set until the educator establishes the learner's needs, when the learner is ready to learn, and how the learner best learns. Learning by the patient, family member, nurses, and other healthcare professionals requires the educator to identify learning approaches and activities based on each individual's learning determinants.

REVIEW QUESTIONS

1. How would you define the term *determinants of learning*?
2. What are four of the seven methods to assess learning needs?
3. What is meant by the term readiness to learn?
4. What are the four types of readiness to learn?
5. What are the components of each type of readiness to learn?
6. What are the six learning style principles that should guide the nurse educator in teaching any audience of learners?
7. Which is the most reliable and valid method to determine someone's learning style?
8. What do each of the eight learning style instruments measure?

CHAPTER 5
DEVELOPMENTAL STAGES OF THE LEARNER

Overview:

In this chapter, the distinct life stages of learners are examined from the perspective of physical, cognitive, and psychosocial development; the role of the nurse in assessment of stage-specific learner needs; the role of the family in the teaching–learning process; and teaching strategies specific to meeting the needs of learners at various developmental stages of life. Although this chapter focuses on the patient as the learner throughout the life span, the stage-specific characteristics of adulthood and the associated teaching principles of adult learning presented can be applied to any audience of older learners, whether the nurse is instructing the general public in the community or teaching continuing education to staff nurses. Emphasis is placed on the learning needs of the adult learner because middle-aged and older adults account for the largest percentage of the patient population.

Learning Outcomes
After completing this chapter, the reader will be able to:
1. Identify the physical, cognitive, and psychosocial characteristics of learners that influence learning at various stages of growth and development.
2. Recognize the role of the nurse as educator in assessing stage-specific learner needs according to maturational levels.
3. Determine the role of the family in patient education.
4. Discuss appropriate teaching strategies effective for learners at different developmental stages.

DEVELOPMENTAL STAGES OF THE LEARNER

The nurse as educator must carefully analyze the features of learners in relation to their developmental stage in life when planning, designing, and implementing an educational program. The more diverse the target audience, the more difficult it is to establish an educational curriculum that meets all of the population's demands. Conversely, the more homogeneous the learner population, the more straightforward the teaching strategy.

I. CHARACTERISTICS OF DEVELOPMENT

The chronological age of a person is simply a relative measure of their physical, cognitive, and psychosocial development stage. Despite the fact that each person is unique, several common developmental trends have been identified as milestones in normal life progression. To completely grasp the behavioral changes that occur in the cognitive, emotional, and psychomotor domains, it is necessary to evaluate the developmental phases as an individual develops from infancy to senescence while dealing with the teaching-learning process. Age, as important as it is in terms of learning readiness, should never be considered in isolation. Experiential history, physical and emotional health status, and personal motivation, as well as several contextual elements such as stress, the surrounding environment, and available support systems, all influence a person's aptitude and readiness to learn. Assume the nurse's role as an educator is to urge students to take charge of their own health. Learners must be considered as a valuable source of information about their health status in this scenario. Before any learning can take place, the nurse must determine how much knowledge the learner already has about the topic being taught. When dealing with a child as a client, new content should be introduced at the proper stages of development and should build on the child's prior knowledge and experiences. When is the best or most appropriate time to instruct the student? The answer is when the learner is ready—what Havighurst (1976) calls the "teachable moment," or the period in time when a learner is most receptive to a teaching setting. It's vital to remember that the nurse as educator isn't required to wait all of the time.

For teachable moments to occur, the instructor must take an interest in and attend to the needs of the student. When determining whether a learner is ready to learn, the nurse educator must consider not only whether an interpersonal relationship has been established, whether prerequisite knowledge and skills have been mastered, and whether the learner is motivated, but also whether the teaching plan is appropriate for the learner's developmental level (Hussey & Hirsh, 1983).

II. THE STAGES OF CHILDHOOD DEVELOPMENT

The art and science of assisting children in learning is known as pedagogy. Developmental theorists and educational psychologists split childhood into stages based on certain patterns of behavior observed during specific stages of growth and development. The table below summarizes the teaching tactics that should be employed in each of the four stages of childhood in relation to the physical, cognitive, and psychosocial maturity levels that indicate learner preparedness. Table 1. Four stages of childhood indicative of learner readiness

Learner	General Characteristics	Teaching Strategies	Nursing Interventions
Infancy–Toddlerhood Approximate age: ➤ Birth–3 years ➤ Cognitive stage: Sensorimotor Psychosocial stage: ➤ Trust vs. mistrust (Birth - 12 months) ➤ Autonomy vs. shame & doubt (1 - 3 years)	✓ Dependent on environment ✓ Needs security ✓ Explores self and environment ✓ Natural curiosity	✓ Orient teaching to caregiver ✓ Use repetition and imitation of information ✓ Stimulate all senses ✓ Provide physical safety and emotional security ✓ Allow play and manipulation of objects	✓ Welcome active involvement ✓ Forge alliances ✓ Encourage physical closeness ✓ Provide detailed information ✓ Answer questions and concerns ✓ Ask for information on child's strengths or limitations and likes or dislikes
Early Childhood Approximate age: ➤ 3-5 years Cognitive stage: ➤ Preoperational Psychosocial stage: ➤ Initiative vs. guilt	✓ Egocentric ✓ Thinking pre-causal, concrete, literal ✓ Believes illness self-caused and punitive ✓ Limited sense of time ✓ Fears bodily injury ✓ Cannot generalize ✓ Animistic thinking (objects possess life or human characteristics)	✓ Use warm, calm approach ✓ Build trust ✓ Use repetition of information ✓ Allow manipulation of objects and equipment ✓ Give care with explanation ✓ Reassure not to blame self ✓ Explain procedures simply and briefly	✓ Welcome active involvement ✓ Forge alliances ✓ Encourage physical closeness ✓ Provide detailed information ✓ Answer questions and concerns ✓ Ask for information on child's strengths/limitations and likes/dislikes

		✓ Centration (focus is on one characteristic of an object) ✓ Separation anxiety ✓ Motivated by curiosity ✓ Active imagination, prone to fears ✓ Play is his/her work\	✓ Provide safe, secure environment ✓ Use positive reinforcement ✓ Encourage questions to reveal perceptions/feelings ✓ Use simple drawings and stories ✓ Use play therapy, with dolls and puppets ✓ Stimulate senses: visual, auditory, tactile, motor	
	Middle and Late Childhood Approximate age: ➢ 6-11 years Cognitive stage: ➢ Concrete operations Psychosocial stage: ➢ Industry vs. inferiority		✓ More realistic and objective ✓ Understands cause and effect ✓ Deductive/inductive reasoning ✓ Wants concrete information ✓ Able to compare objects and events ✓ Variable rates of physical growth ✓ Reasons syllogistically ✓ Understands seriousness and consequences of actions ✓ Subject-centered focus ✓ Immediate orientation	✓ Encourage independence and active participation ✓ Be honest, allay fears ✓ Use logical explanation ✓ Allow time to ask questions ✓ Use analogies to make invisible processes real ✓ Establish role models ✓ Relate care to other children's experiences; compare procedures ✓ Use subject-centered focus ✓ Use play therapy ✓ Provide group activities ✓ Use drawings, models, dolls, painting, audio- and videotapes	✓ Welcome active involvement ✓ Forge alliances ✓ Encourage physical closeness ✓ Provide detailed information ✓ Answer questions and concerns ✓ Ask for information on child's strengths/limitations and likes/dislikes
	Adolescence Approximate age: ➢ 12-19 years Cognitive stage: ➢ Formal operations Psychosocial stage ➢ Identity vs. role confusion	✓ Abstract, hypothetical thinking ✓ Can build on past learning ✓ Reasons by logic and understands scientific principles ✓ Future orientation ✓ Motivated by desire for social acceptance ✓ Peer group important ✓ Intense personal preoccupation, appearance extremely important (imaginary audience)	✓ Establish trust, authenticity ✓ Know their agenda ✓ Address fears/concerns about outcomes of illness ✓ Identify control focus ✓ Include in plan of care ✓ Use peers for support and influence ✓ Negotiate changes ✓ Focus on details ✓ Make information meaningful to life ✓ Ensure confidentiality and privacy	✓ Explore emotional and financial support ✓ Determine goals and expectations ✓ Assess stress levels ✓ Respect values and norms ✓ Determine role responsibilities and relationships ✓ Engage in 1:1 teaching without parents present, but with adolescent's permission inform

		✓ Feels invulnerable, invincible/immune to natural laws (personal fable)	✓ Arrange group sessions ✓ Use audiovisuals, role play, contracts, reading materials ✓ Provide for experimentation and flexibility	family of content covered
Young Adulthood Approximate age: ➢ 20-40 years Cognitive stage: ➢ Formal operations Psychosocial stage: ➢ Intimacy vs. isolation		✓ Autonomous ✓ Self-directed ✓ Uses personal experiences to enhance or interfere with learning ✓ Intrinsic motivation ✓ Able to analyze critically ✓ Makes decisions about personal, occupational, and social roles ✓ Competency-based learner	✓ Use problem-centered focus ✓ Draw on meaningful experiences ✓ Focus on immediacy of application ✓ Encourage active participation ✓ Allow to set own pace, be self-directed ✓ Organize material ✓ Recognize social role ✓ Apply new knowledge through role playing and hands-on practice	✓ Explore emotional, financial, and physical support system ✓ Assess motivational level for involvement ✓ Identify potential obstacles and stressors
MIDDLE-AGED ADULTHOOD Approximate age: 41-64 years Cognitive stage: Formal operations Psychosocial stage: Generativity vs. self-absorption and stagnation		✓ Sense of self well-developed ✓ Concerned with physical changes ✓ At peak in career ✓ Explores alternative lifestyles ✓ Reflects on contributions to family and society ✓ Reexamines goals and values ✓ Questions achievements and successes ✓ Has confidence in abilities ✓ Desires to modify unsatisfactory aspects of life	✓ x Focus on maintaining independence and reestablishing normal life patterns ✓ Assess positive and negative past experiences with learning ✓ Assess potential sources of stress caused by midlife crisis issues ✓ Provide information to coincide with life concerns and problems	✓ Explore emotional, financial, and physical support system ✓ Assess motivational level for involvement ✓ Identify potential obstacles and stressors
Older Adulthood Approximate age: ➢ 65 years and over Cognitive stage: ➢ Formal operations Psychosocial stage: ➢ Ego integrity vs. despair		<u>Cognitive changes:</u> ✓ Decreased ability to think abstractly, process information ✓ Decreased short-term memory ✓ Increased reaction time ✓ Increased test anxiety ✓ Stimulus persistence (afterimage)	✓ Use concrete examples ✓ Build on past life experiences ✓ Make information relevant and meaningful ✓ Present one concept at a time ✓ Allow time for processing/response (slow pace)	✓ Involve principal caregivers ✓ Encourage participation ✓ Provide resources for support (respite care) ✓ Assess coping mechanisms ✓ Provide written instructions for reinforcement

	✓ Focuses on past life experiences **Sensory/motor deficits:** ✓ Auditory changes ✓ Hearing loss, especially high-pitched tones, consonants (S, Z, T, F, and G), and rapid speech ✓ Visual changes ✓ Farsighted (needs glasses to read) ✓ Lenses become opaque (glare problem) ✓ Smaller pupil size (decreased visual adaptation to darkness) ✓ Decreased peripheral perception ✓ Yellowing of lenses (distorts low-tone colors: blue, green, violet) ✓ Distorted depth perception ✓ Fatigue/decreased energy levels ✓ Pathophysiology (chronic illness) **Psychosocial changes:** ✓ Decreased risk taking ✓ Selective learning ✓ Intimidated by formal learning	✓ Use repetition and reinforcement of information ✓ Avoid written exams ✓ Use verbal exchange and coaching ✓ Establish retrieval plan (use one or several clues) ✓ Encourage active involvement ✓ Keep explanations brief ✓ Use analogies to illustrate abstract information ✓ Speak slowly, distinctly ✓ Use low-pitched tones ✓ Avoid shouting ✓ Use visual aids to supplement verbal instruction ✓ Avoid glares, use soft white light ✓ Provide suffcient light ✓ Use white backgrounds and black print ✓ Use large letters and well-spaced print ✓ Avoid color coding with pastel blues, greens, purples, and yellows ✓ Increase safety precautions/provide safe environment ✓ Ensure accessibility and fit of prostheses (i.e., glasses, hearing aid) ✓ Keep sessions short ✓ Provide for frequent rest periods ✓ Allow for extra time to perform ✓ Establish realistic short-term goals ✓ Give time to reminisce ✓ Identify and present pertinent material ✓ Use informal teaching sessions	✓ Provide anticipatory problem solving (what happens if …)

			✓ Demonstrate relevance of information to daily life ✓ Assess resources ✓ Make learning positive ✓ Identify past positive experiences ✓ Integrate new behaviors with formerly established ones	

I. THE DEVELOPMENTAL STAGES OF ADULTHOOD

Andragogy, the term coined by Knowles (1990) to describe his theory of adult learning, is the art and science of helping adults learn. Education within this framework is more learner-centered and less teacher-centered; that is, instead of one party imparting knowledge on another, the power relationship between the educator and the adult learner is much more horizontal (Milligan, 1997).

The following basic assumptions about Knowles's framework have major implications for planning, implementing, and evaluating teaching programs for adults as the individual matures:

1. His or her self-concept moves from being a dependent personality to being an independent, self-directed human being.
2. He or she accumulates a growing reservoir of previous experience that serves as a rich resource for learning.
3. Readiness to learn becomes increasingly oriented to the developmental tasks of social roles.
4. The perspective of time changes from one of postponed application of knowledge to one of immediate application; there is a shift in orientation of learning from being subject centered to problem centered.

Table 2. Summary of Adult Learning Principles

ADULTS LEARN BEST WHEN:	
Principle #1	Learning is related to an immediate need, problem, or deficit. Learning is voluntary and self-initiated.
Principle #2	Learning is person-centered and problem-centered. Learning is self-controlled and self-directed.
Principle #3	The role of the teacher is one of facilitator. Information and assignments are pertinent.
Principle #4	New material draws on past experiences and is related to something the learner already knows. The threat to self is reduced to a minimum in the educational situation.
Principle #5	The learner is able to participate actively in the learning process. The learner is able to learn in a group.
Principle #6	The nature of the learning activity changes frequently. Learning is reinforced by application and prompt feedback.
Principle #7	Learning is related to an immediate need, problem, or deficit. Learning is voluntary and self-initiated.
Principle #8	Learning is person-centered and problem-centered. Learning is self-controlled and self-directed.
Principle #9	The role of the teacher is one of facilitator. Information and assignments are pertinent.
Principle #10	New material draws on past experiences and is related to something the learner already knows. The threat to self is reduced to a minimum in the educational situation.
Principle #11	The learner is able to participate actively in the learning process. The learner is able to learn in a group.
Principle #12	The nature of the learning activity changes frequently. Learning is reinforced by application and prompt feedback.

SOURCE: Adapted from Burgireno, J. (1985). Maximizing learning in the adult with SCI. *Rehabilitation Nursing*, 10(5), 20–21.

II. **THE ROLE OF THE FAMILY IN PATIENT EDUCATION**

One of the important determinants impacting patient treatment outcomes is the role of the family (Reeber, 1992). The key goals of incorporating family members in the care delivery and decision-making process in patient education are to reduce stress associated with hospitalization, lower healthcare costs, and successfully educate the client for self-care management outside of the healthcare setting. The patient's emotional, physical, and social needs are met by family caregivers (Gilroth, 1990). Involving family members in the teaching–

learning process ensures that both the client and the nurse educator benefit. Healthcare workers are responsible for aiding patients and their families in gaining the knowledge and skills needed to satisfy their continuing healthcare needs (Hartman & Kochar, 1994). Enhancement of family roles and increased knowledge on the side of the family has favorable consequences for both the learner and the teacher. Clients gain more satisfaction and freedom in self-care, and nurses gain more job satisfaction and personal gratification by assisting clients in reaching their full potential and achieving successful outcomes (Barnes, 1995).

SUMMARY

To individualize the approach to education in fulfilling the needs and wants of learners and their families, it is critical to grasp the distinct and different duties connected with each developmental stage. The assessment of physical, cognitive, and psychosocial maturation within each developmental period is critical in defining the teaching-learning modalities to be applied. In many respects, the younger learner differs from the adult learner. Dependency, level of participation, pace of and learning ability, as well as situational and emotional barriers to learning, differ considerably between developmental stages. The subject-centered nature of children's readiness to learn is heavily influenced by their physical, cognitive, and psychosocial maturity. Adult motivation to learn is problem-oriented and more focused on psychosocial tasks connected to work, family, and community duties and expectations. To be effective, the nurse as educator must create a learning environment by providing material at the learner's level, soliciting participation and feedback, and determining whether parental and/or peer involvement is acceptable or essential. In light of the learner's developmental stage, nurses, as the primary source of health education, must assess what needs to be taught, when to teach, how to teach, and who should be the focus of teaching.

CONTENT EVALUATION

The evaluation after the end of this chapter will be done through a take-home quiz, which the students must answer. Citations from other sources must be referenced by way of footnotes. Each paper will go through a plagiarism checker to ensure that none of the answers are copy pasted. The output shall be submitted by way of e-mail, and shall form part of the student's overall grade.

REVIEW QUESTIONS

1. What are the seven (7) stages of development?
2. What is the definition of *pedagogy, andragogy,* and *gerogogy*?
3. What are the salient characteristics at each stage of development that influence the ability to learn?
4. What are three (3) main teaching strategies for each stage of development?
5. How do people you know in each stage of development compare with what you have learned about physical, cognitive, and psychosocial characteristics at the various develop- mental stages?
6. What is the role of the family in the teaching and learning process in each stage of development?
7. How does the role of the nurse vary when teaching individuals at different stages of development?

CHAPTER 6
MOTIVATION, COMPLIANCE, AND HEALTH BEHAVIORS OF THE LEARNER

Overview:

This chapter discusses the concepts of motivation and compliance as they relate to the learning situation with a focus on health behaviors. The discussion includes factors such as assessment of motivation, obstacles and facilitating factors for motivation and compliance, and motivational axioms. An overview and comparison of selected models of health behaviors are presented, emphasizing the role of the nurse as an educator in health promotion.

Learning Outcomes

After completing this chapter, the student will be able to:

1. Define the terms *motivation*, *compliance*, and *adherence* relevant to behaviors of the learner.
2. Discuss motivation and compliance concepts and theories.
3. Identify incentives and obstacles that affect motivation to learn.
4. Discuss axioms of motivation relevant to learning.
5. Assess levels of learner motivation
6. Outline strategies that facilitate motivation and improve compliance.
7. Compare and contrast selected health behavior frameworks and their influence on learning.

8. Recognize the unique sub-roles of the nurse as educator in health promotion.

MOTIVATION, COMPLIANCE, AND HEALTH BEHAVIORS OF THE LEARNER

Many health behavior models use the notions of compliance and incentive, either implicitly or explicitly. This chapter covers these concepts as they relate to the learner's health behaviors, as well as providing an overview of selected theories and models to consider during the teaching-learning process. As an educator, the nurse must grasp what elements support or hinder knowledge acquisition and application, as well as what motivates the learner to learn. Health behaviors and outcomes are influenced by a variety of factors. Knowledge does not ensure that the learner will engage in health-promoting actions or attain the desired results. If the learner is not understood in the context of complicated elements related with compliance and motivation, even the most well-thought-out educational program or plan of care will fail to attain the specified goals.

I. MOTIVATION

Motivation is derived from the Latin word movere, which meaning "to set in motion." Motivation has been defined as a psychological force that propels a person to take action (Haggard, 1989), as well as a learner's willingness to embrace learning, with preparedness as proof of motivation (Redman, 2001). It is the product of both internal and external forces, according to Kort (1987), rather than the effect of external manipulation alone. Movement in the direction of meeting a need or achieving a goal is implicit in motivation. [1]

Factors that influence motivation. Motivating factors can act as both incentives and roadblocks to achieving desired actions. The nurse as educator faces a difficulty in both establishing rewards and removing barriers to motivation. The educator can influence the learner's cognitive (thinking processes), affective (emotions and feelings), social, and psychomotor (behavioral) domains by acting as a motivating facilitator or blocker.

In order to be effective, motivational incentives must be examined in the context of the individual. What may serve as a motivator for one student may serve as a deterrent for another. A student who is assigned to work with an elderly woman, for example, may be motivated if the student values older people. Another student could be demotivated by the same emotional area since earlier interactions with elderly women, such as a grandma, were unsatisfactory. There are three basic categories of facilitating or blocking elements that determine motivation to learn, which are not mutually exclusive:

a) Personal characteristics, which include the learner's physical, developmental, and psychological characteristics.

b) Environmental factors, such as the physical and psychological environment

c) Learner connection systems, such as those between a significant other, a family, a community, and a teacher and a student.

Axioms of Motivation

Axioms are premises that are used to understand a phenomenon. As an educator, the nurse must be aware of the factors that influence the learner's motivation. Axioms of motivation are rules that set the tone for motivation. They are: (1) optimal anxiety, (2) learner readiness, (3) realistic goal setting, (4) learner satisfaction/success, and (5) discourse that reduces or maintains uncertainty.

a) Optimal Anxiety Level - Learning is most effective when there is a reasonable level of anxiety. One's ability to observe, focus attention, learn, and adapt is operational in this optimal learning state (Peplau, 1979)

b) Learner Willingness - Motivation is influenced by the desire to achieve a goal and the readiness to learn. The learner's desire cannot be forced. External pressures, on the other hand, can have a significant impact on it, and the nurse's role as an educator can help to encourage it.

c) Realistic Goals - Individuals will work toward realistic goals that are within their reach, sensible, and achievable. Goals that are out of reach are both annoying and ineffective. Unrealistic goals, along with the loss of crucial time, might lead to a learner's decision to "give up."

d) Learner Satisfaction/Success - Success motivates the learner. Success gives one a sense of accomplishment and boosts one's self-esteem. Success and self-esteem rise in a cyclical process, propelling the learner toward goal achievement. Motivation is increased when a student feels good about their small victories. [1]

e) Uncertainty Reduction or Maintenance - In a learning scenario, uncertainty (together with certainty) can be a motivating force. Individuals have constant internal conversations that can minimize or maintain uncertainty. When it comes to changing one's health, a discourse that examines ambiguity is common: "If I stop smoking, my chances of acquiring lung cancer will be reduced." When the likely outcome of health behaviors is more unknown, however, behaviors such as "I am not sure that I need this operation because the survival percentages are the same for those who had this surgery and those who did not" may be maintained.

II. MANAGEMENT AND COMPLIANCE

Submission or submitting to established aims is referred to as compliance. It has a manipulative or authoritative undertone when defined as such, with the healthcare professional or educator perceived as the traditional authority and the consumer or student as submissive. [3]

Noncompliance refers to a person's unwillingness to follow a set of instructions.

The authoritative feature of compliance implies that the educator is attempting to regulate, at least in part, the learner's decision-making. By employing words like mutual contracting (Steckel, 1982) or consensual regimen, some compliance models have attempted to balance the issue of control (Fink, 1976).

The concepts of locus of control (Rotter, 1954) and health locus of control are two ways to look at the issue of control in the learning setting (Wallston, Wallston, & DeVellis, 1978). Individuals can be classified as "internals," whose health behavior is self-directed, or "externals," in which others are perceived as more powerful in influencing health outcomes, based on objective measurement. [1]

Internals feel they have control over their own destiny, but externals believe fate is a powerful external force that controls life's trajectory. "Osteoporosis runs in my family, and it will 'catch up' with me," an outsider might say. "Although my family has a history of osteoporosis, I will have the necessary screenings, maintain an appropriate diet, and engage in weight-bearing activity to prevent or control this problem," an internal may state. [4]

III. THE LEARNER'S HEALTH ATTITUDES

Motivation and compliance are topics that are related to the learner's health behaviors. As an educator, the nurse emphasizes health education as well as expected health habits. Health behavior frameworks are blueprints that act as educational aids for nurses. They can be used to sustain or encourage desired patient behaviors. As a result, knowing models and theories that describe, explain, or predict health behaviors will broaden the spectrum of health-promoting measures available to the nurse educator. The ideas inherent in each of these frameworks can be used to either facilitate motivation or increase compliance with a health regimen once they are understood.

A summary of various models and theories:

A. Model of Health Belief

The Health Belief Model is based on the idea that three key interacting components can be used to predict health behavior: individual perceptions, modifying influences, and likelihood of action [5].

B. Model of Health Promotion

The Health Promotion Model is more focused on health promotion than disease prevention. It focuses on realizing one's health potential and raising one's level of well-being through approach behaviors rather than disease avoidance.

Self-Efficacy Theory (theory of self-efficacy)

The Self-Efficacy Theory, which was developed from a social-cognitive perspective, is based on a person's expectations in relation to a given course of action (Bandura, 1986). It is a predictive theory in the sense that it is concerned with the assumption that a given behavior can be accomplished. Expected outcomes are preceded by the belief in competency and capability in relation to specific acts.

Model of Change Stages (D)

This approach was established in the field of psychology to deal with addictive and troublesome behaviors. Precontemplation, contemplation, preparation, action, maintenance, and termination are the six stages of transformation identified by Prochaska (1996).

1. Individuals in the precontemplation stage have no immediate plans to change. Simple observations, confrontation, or consciousness-raising are examples of strategies.

2. Contemplation stage - people accept or recognize that they have a problem and begin to actively consider how to solve it. Increased awareness-raising is one of the strategies.

3. The planning stage - folks are planning to act within a month's time range. A clear and precise action plan is part of a strategy.

4. Action - there is a change in conduct that is overt or obvious. Commitment to the change, self-reward, countering (substitute behaviors), building a welcoming environment, and supporting connections are among the tactics used at this stage. [5]

5. Maintenance - this is the most difficult stage to complete and can span anywhere from six months to a lifetime. Overconfidence, constant temptation, and relapse self-blame are all common obstacles at this point. This stage's strategies are the same as those used in the action stage.

6. Termination - this occurs when the problem is no longer enticing. However, according to some specialists, there is no termination; just maintenance becomes less diligent.

E. Reasoned Action Theory

The Theory of Reasoned Action is founded on the assumption that humans are rational decision makers who use whatever information they have at their disposal. This theory does not include attitudes toward people; rather, it focuses on the projected behavior.

The Theory of Reasoned Action is valuable in forecasting health behaviors, especially for educators interested in understanding the attitudinal context in which behaviors are likely to change. When constructing educational programs pertaining to the purpose to modify a certain health behavior, nurses as educators must examine beliefs, attitudinal factors, and subjective standards.

F. MODEL OF PRECEDE-PROCEEDING

The PRECEDE-PROCEED Model was born out of an epidemiological approach to health promotion in the hopes of reducing the number of people dying from the primary causes of death (Green & Kreuter, 1999). Green, Kreuter, Deeds, and Partridge established the PRECEDE paradigm, which stands for Predisposing, Reinforcing, and Enabling Constructs in Educational Diagnosis and Evaluation (1980). Green and Kreuter (1999) modified the model by adding a second component called PROCEED (Policy, Regulatory, and Organizational Constructs in Educational and Environmental Development), which stands for Policy, Regulatory, and Organizational Constructs in Educational and Environmental Development.

The model's foundation is health education, which is defined as "any combination of learning experiences meant to facilitate voluntary acts beneficial to health" (Green & Kreuter, 1999, p. 27). Green and Kreuter go on to say that the goal of health education is to "predispose, empower, and encourage voluntary behavior beneficial to the health of individuals, groups, or communities" through learning experiences (p. 506).

I. MODEL SELECTION FOR HEALTH EDUCATION

Models for instructional usage can be chosen based on (1) similarities and differences, (2) agreement with model conceptualizations by nurses as educators, and (3) functional utility.

Models' Similarities and Dissimilarities

Models may appear to be so similar that choosing one over the other is a moot point, or they may appear to be so dissimilar that one is improper for a given educational goal.

The Health Belief Model and the Health Promotion Model are similar, according to a comparison of the different frameworks. The discrepancies can be seen in the basic assumptions and outcomes of the models. The Health Belief Model places a premium on illness vulnerability and the likelihood of taking preventative action, whereas the Health Promotion Model places a premium on health potential and health-promoting behaviors.

The Self-Efficacy Theory and the Theory of Reasoned Action are similar in that they both focus on behavioral predictions or expectations. Because the theories are more linear in conceptualization, they lend themselves more easily to less sophisticated model testing than either the Health Belief Model or the Health Promotion Model. The ability to target the results of educational programs may be aided by the specificity of actions. [5]

In the sense that all of these models focus on intent, the Stages of Change Model is comparable to the Self-Efficacy Theory and the Theory of Reasoned Action. The Stages of Change Model, on the other hand, is more basic and does not take into account human qualities or experiences. It differs from the Self-Efficacy Theory and the Theory of Reasoned Action in that interventions are guided by stages and strategies for transformation within each step.

The Health Belief Model, Health Promotion Model, Self-Efficacy Theory, and Theory of Reasoned Action are all similar in that they accept both internal and external elements that can affect health behaviors, such as experiences, perceptions, or beliefs. These frameworks also take into account the multifaceted character, complexity, and likelihood of health behaviors. This perspective is broadened by the PRECEDE-PROCEED model, which includes aggregates and populations.

All of the models recognize the relevance of the patient's input into health-related decision-making. The distinctions are based on the patient's attention, the relative importance of modifying factors, behavior specificity, and outcomes.

The Therapeutic Alliance Model is the most dissimilar. Its simplicity and parsimony are its assets, despite its limited reach. When it comes to education, the educator–learner relationship is the most important aspect. When dealing with potentially frustrating patient education situations like noncompliance, Hochbaum (1980) observed that frustrated patient educators "are unable to understand the apparently irrational and self-destructive action of their patients, and sometimes throw their hands up in despair, bedeviled by the seeming irrationality of the patient's behavior.." (p. 7). The Therapeutic Alliance Model can help you understand your client as a learner.

Educator Agreement with Model Conceptualizations

Nurses as educators have belief systems, which may or may not agree with some of the tenets of each of the models presented. Therefore, the choice of a model can be based on the educator's level of agreement with salient factors in each framework.

Functional Utility of Models

Model selection for educational purposes can also be based on functional utility. Questions to be asked to determine functional utility are as follows:

a) Who is the target learner?
b) What is the focus of the learning?
c) When is the optimal time?
d) Where is the process to be carried out?

I. THE SUB-ROLES OF NURSE AS EDUCATOR IN HEALTH PROMOTION

Nurses, as educators, may help people live healthier lives. An integrated approach to molding the learner's health behaviors is possible by combining content relevant to the field of nursing, knowledge from educational theories, and health behavior models. Facilitator of change, contractor, organizer, and evaluator are all sub-roles of the nurse as educator.

A. Change Facilitator - The nurse's purpose as an educator is, of course, to promote health. This endeavour necessitates the use of health education and promotion. At the same time, the nurse's role as an educator is critical in facilitating change. When learning is viewed as a nursing intervention, it must be examined in conjunction with other nursing interventions that promote change. Explaining, analyzing, separating complicated abilities, demonstrating, practicing, asking questions, and providing closure are all effective ways to facilitate change in the learning context, according to DeTornay and Thompson (1987).

B. Contractor - Contracting has long been a popular way to make learning more convenient. Learning objectives can be defined and promoted through informal or formal contracts. Educational contracting, like the nursing process, entails defining mutual goals, devising an agreed-upon plan of action, assessing the plan, and deriving alternatives.

C. Organizer - The nurse as educator is responsible for the organization of the learning environment, including the management of resources and space, the sequential organizing of content from simple to complicated, and the determination of subject matter priority. Learning difficulties are reduced when learning materials are organized (Haggard, 1989). To facilitate the learning process and boost motivation to learn, attendance at educational programs or individual sessions can be planned around the target learner as well as significant people.

D. Evaluator - Educational initiatives, like other healthcare undertakings, must be held accountable to the learner or patient. Evaluation in the form of outcomes ensures this accountability. Self-assessment, patient evaluation, organization evaluation, and peer evaluation are all notions that have been around for a long time. All forms of learning include evaluative procedures. The nurse's position as an educator has been questioned. The distinction between patient education and patient teaching is made by Luker and Caress (1989), who state that the former is the responsibility of the clinical specialist. They also point out that not all nurses are equipped to educate patients. The impact of a specialist approach to education on health outcomes as well as professional role must be examined. In the end, the evaluative measure of learning is the application of information that enhances the health of individuals, families, groups, or communities.

SUMMARY

A review of motivation and compliance ideas, an assessment of learner motivation level, identification of incentives and impediments that affect motivation and compliance, and a discussion of axioms of motivation related to learning were all important parts of this chapter. Furthermore, various health behavior frameworks and their impact on learning have been compared and contrasted, specific incentive and compliance tactics have been detailed, and the nurse's unique role as educator in influencing learner motivation and compliance has been addressed. The basis for change in health behaviors is laid when information is conveyed, accepted, and applied. A barrier to health is removed when people are motivated and believe they can make a difference in their own lives.

REVIEW QUESTIONS

1. How are the terms *motivation, compliance,* and *adherence* defined?
2. How do the terms defined in Question 1 relate to one another?
3. What are the three (3) major motivational factors?
4. Which axioms (premises) are involved in promoting motivation of the learner?
5. What are the six (6) parameters for a comprehensive motivational assessment of the learner?
6. What are the six (6) major models or theories used to describe, explain,

or predict health behaviors?

7. Which models/theories are used to facilitate motivation and which ones are used to pro- mote compliance to a therapeutic healthcare regimen?

8. What are the basic concepts particular to each model or theory?

9. What are the similarities and differences between the models with respect to who is the target audience, what is the focus of the learning, and where is the education process to be carried out?

10. What are the sub-roles of the nurse in shaping health behaviors of the learner?

CHATER 7
GENDER, SOCIOECONOMIC, AND CULTURAL ATTRIBUTES OF THE LEARNER

Overview:

This chapter examines how individuals respond differently to healthcare interventions by looking at gender-related differences resulting from heredity or social conditioning that affect how the brain functions for learning, the impact of the learner's environment from a socioeconomic standpoint, and the significant effects cultural norms have on learners' behaviors from the persuasion perspective. Additionally, approaches for cultural evaluation and care planning are discussed. This chapter also discusses how to prepare nurses for diverse patient care and how to deal with stereotyping.

Outcomes of Learning:

The student will be able to do the following after finishing this chapter:
1. Recognize the role of socioeconomic factors in impacting one's health condition and habits.
2. Examine cultural assessment from the standpoint of various care models.
3. Make recommendations for teaching tactics tailored to the requirements of students from each of the four historically underrepresented groups.
4. Consider how transcultural nursing might be used as a framework for serving the educational requirements of diverse ethnic groups.

5. Define stereotyping, the risks associated with it, and ways to avoid stereotyped behavior.

THE LEARNER'S GENDER, SOCIOECONOMIC, AND CULTURAL ATTRIBUTES

Gender, financial status, and cultural background all have an impact on a learner's propensity to respond to and utilize the teaching–learning scenario. Nurse educators have paid very little attention to two of these factors: gender and socioeconomic position. Cultural and ethnic diversity, the third element, has been the subject of much research in recent years in terms of its implications on learning. When creating and implementing education programs to address the requirements of an increasingly diverse group of learners, it is critical to understand diversity, particularly differences among learners related to gender, socioeconomics, and culture.

I. DIFFERENCES BETWEEN MEN AND WOMEN

In events affecting all aspects of life, there are sex disparities in how males and females act, respond, and perform. In human relationships, women's intuition tends to pick up subtle tones of voice and facial expressions, whereas men's intuition is less sensitive to these communication cues; in navigation, women have difficulty finding their way, whereas men appear to have a better sense of direction; and in cognition, females excel in languages and verbalization, while men demonstrate stronger sp Scientists are beginning to assume that gender differences in the brain have as much to do with brain biology as they do with upbringing (Gorman, 1992). In terms of brain functioning, gender disparities are likely due to a combination of heredity and environmental influences. The list of cognitive skills and gender-related differences for each ability is as follows (Gage & Berliner, 1998):

A. General intelligence: Various research have come up with conflicting results when it comes to whether males and females have different levels of general intelligence. On broad IQ tests, no significant disparities between men and women have been discovered.

B. Verbal ability: Girls learn to talk, form sentences, and employ a larger vocabulary than boys. Girls also speak more eloquently, read earlier, and do consistently better on spelling and grammar examinations.

C. Mathematical ability: There appear to be no gender-related differences in math aptitude during the preschool years. Males, on the other hand, show signs of excelling in mathematical reasoning by the end of elementary school, and the disparities in arithmetic aptitude between boys and girls become even higher in high school.

D. Spatial ability: Males regularly outperform females on the capacity to recognize a rotating figure, discern a shape embedded in another figure, and accurately recreate a three-dimensional object. Of all the various gender-related disparities in intellectual activity, males' spatial ability is consistently higher than females', and this is most likely due to genetics.

E. Problem solving: Research into the complex concepts of problem solving, creativity, analytical ability, and cognitive styles has yielded mixed results in terms of gender differences. Men are more likely to try new ways to problem solving and to be "field independent" in some learning tasks, which means they are less influenced by irrelevant cues and more focused on common aspects. In risk-taking circumstances, men also display more curiosity and less conservatism than women. Women, on the other hand, are better at problem-solving than men in the domain of human interactions.

F. Academic achievement: Girls consistently outperform boys in school, particularly at the elementary school level. Girls' academic performance is more consistent and less variable than boys'.

G. Aggression: In most societies, males of all ages are more aggressive than females. The role of testosterone, a gender-specific hormone, is being explored as a possible cause of males' greater violent behavior.

H. Dependence and conformity: Females have been proven to be more compliant and more swayed by suggestion than males. However, due to gender biases in some research, these findings have been questioned.

I. Emotional adjustment: While both boys and girls have similar emotional stability in childhood, there are variances in how emotional difficulties develop. According to some data, teenage and adult females experience higher neurotic symptoms than males. Still, this trend could be explained by how society defines mental health in ways that align with male roles, or by the fact that mental health exams are typically devised by males and hence may be biased.

J. Ideals and life goals: Men have traditionally had a stronger interest in scientific, mathematical, mechanical, and physically active vocations, as well as stronger theoretical, economic, and political values. Women have a stronger aesthetic, social sense, and religious values, and have a tendency to select literary, social service, and clerical vocations.

K. Accomplishment orientation: Women are more likely than men to demonstrate achievement motivation in social skills and social relationships, whereas men are more likely to succeed in intellectual or competitive pursuits. This disparity is assumed to be due to sex-role expectations that are instilled in children at a young age.

Teaching Techniques

Nurses must become aware of the extent to which gender-related social and hereditary disparities affect health-seeking behaviors and influence individual health needs as health educators. Nurses must be aware of the cognitive and personality factors that influence how men and women learn, when they learn, what they are best at learning, and what they are most interested in learning. As previously said, males and females have distinct orientations, learning styles, and levels of success when it comes to communicating and learning in some areas. Men and women belong to separate social cultures. They express themselves through varied symbols, belief systems, and methods, much like different ethnic groups have distinctive cultures. Nurse educators are encouraged to employ a variety of teaching styles in order to avoid perpetuating gender stereotypes in teaching and learning.

I. **SOCIOECONOMIC DIFFERENCES**

Socioeconomic status (SES), in addition to gender differences, influences the teaching-learning process. SES is considered to be the single most important determinant of health in our society (Pappas et al., 1993). SES or socioeconomic class is an aspect of diversity that must be addressed in the context of education and in the process of teaching and learning.

Social and economic levels of individuals have been found to be significant variables affecting health status and in determining health behaviors (Pappas et al., 1993) Individuals who have higher incomes and are better educated live longer and healthier lives than those who are of low income and poorly educated.

Teaching Strategies

Educational interventions by nurses for those who are socially and economically deprived have the potential for yielding short-term benefits in meeting these individuals' immediate healthcare needs.

Nurse educators must be aware of the probable effects of low SES on an individual's ability to learn as a result of suboptimal cognitive functioning, poor academic achievement, low literacy, high susceptibility to illness, and disintegration of social support systems. Low-income people are at greater risk for these factors that can interfere with learning, but one cannot assume that every- one at the poverty or near-poverty level is equally influenced by these threats to their well-being. To avoid stereotyping, each individual or family must be assessed to determine his or her particular strengths and weaknesses for learning. In this way, teaching strategies unique to particular circumstances can be designed to assist socioeconomically deprived individuals in meeting their needs for health care.

II. <u>CULTURAL DIFFERENCES</u>

Nurses will need to be well-versed in the cultural values and beliefs of certain ethnic groups, as well as be cognizant of individual behaviors and preferences, to keep up with a society that is becoming increasingly culturally diverse (Price & Cordell, 1994).

Methods for Providing Culturally Sensitive Care

Given our fast changing world and people's greater geographical mobility, our healthcare system and educational institutions must adjust by shifting from a dominating monocultural, ethnocentric focus to a more multicultural, transcultural orientation.

According to studies, health practitioners are frequently unaware of the numerous aspects that influence patients' reactions to health care. Six cultural phenomena must be considered while doing a nursing assessment: communication, personal space, social structure, time, environmental control, and biological variances (Anderson,1990). Price and Cordell (1994) proposed a four-step process to assist nurses in providing culturally sensitive patient education:

1. Make changes to the client's instruction based on the information gathered in the previous step.
2. Identify the Client's Adaptation
3. Knowledge of the Client's Culture
4. Investigate Personal Culture

Andrews (1992) proposed three ways for the nursing profession to pursue in order to prepare its future practitioners:

1. Nursing professionals from a variety of ethnic origins should be employed and promoted in greater numbers in clinical practice settings. Continuing education programs are needed to raise staff nurses' awareness of their own culturally based values, beliefs, and practices, as well as to expand their knowledge of culture-specific health-related beliefs and practices of others they are likely to encounter within their specialty areas of practice.

2. Nurse educators with formal, in-depth training in transcultural, cross-cultural nursing and perspectives from allied disciplines such as anthropology and sociology are needed to put in more concerted effort in academic settings. Culture-logical evaluation, bio-cultural variations in health and illness, and cultural differences in communication, religious views, diet, elements of aging, and other topics must all be addressed in the classroom. Teaching–learning tactics that take into account the cultural background and situation of the client (Ander- son, 1987, 1990).

3. Cross-cultural studies are required in both basic and applied research domains within the field of research. Cross-cultural studies, the majority of

which rely heavily on qualitative research methodologies, should be fostered by funding agencies and private organizations.

Cultural Analysis

A. The Nurse–Client Negotiations Model was created to aid in cultural assessment and care planning for culturally diverse individuals. The Nurse–Client Negotiations Model is a framework for paying attention to both the nurse's and the client's cultures. Aside from the professional culture, each nurse has his or her own personal ideas and values, which may or may not be completely recognized by the nursing. Nurses' interactions with patients and families may be influenced by their views and values.

B. Campinha-Bacote (1995) suggested the Culturally Competent Paradigm of Care as another model for undertaking a complete and sensitive cultural evaluation.

A set of congruent behaviors, attitudes, and policies that enable a system, agency, or professional to perform effectively in a cross-cultural scenario is defined as cultural competency. Cultural competency is viewed as a continuous process with four components in this model: cultural awareness, cultural knowledge, cultural skill, and cultural encounter.

• Cultural awareness is the process of becoming sensitive to encounters with people from various cultures; it involves nurses to analyze their preconceptions and biases toward people from other cultures.

• Cultural knowledge is the process by which nurses gain a foundation in many cultural worldviews through education.

• The process of learning how to conduct an appropriate cultural evaluation is referred to as cultural skill.

• Cultural encounter promotes nurses to engage in cross-cultural interactions with clients from various cultural backgrounds in the workplace. If one is to provide culturally appropriate nursing care, all four components must be present.

Interventions in Teaching and General Assessment

The nurse in the role of educator must use universal skills such as developing rapport, assessing willingness to learn, and using active listening to analyze and comprehend problems to conduct successful teaching interventions.

The way a sick person is defined and treated is also influenced by culture. Some cultures, for example, think that once symptoms fade away, disease is no longer present. This concept can be troublesome for those who are suffering from an acute sickness like a streptococcal infection, where a one- or two-day course of antibiotic therapy cures throat pain. It's also a concern for someone who suffers from a chronic ailment that goes through periods of remission or exacerbation. Because culture is such an important part in cross-cultural education, readiness to learn must also be judged from that perspective.

Regardless of the client's cultural orientation, the following specific assessment guidelines should be used: (Anderson, 1987)

1. Pay attention to the relationships between the patient and family members, as well as amongst family members. Determine who makes the decisions, how they are made, who is the primary caregiver, what kind of care is provided, and what foods and other items are important to the patient and family.

2. Pay attention to the patient. Learn about the patient's desires, how they differ from the family's desires, and how they differ from what you believe is appropriate.

3. Think about your communication skills and routines. Be mindful of nonverbal behaviors and etiquette of interaction that the patient and family may find acceptable or objectionable, the patient's native language, which may differ from your own, and speaking manners (tempo of speech, expressions used) that can help or hinder understanding.

4. Look into local conventions or taboos. Observe actions and inquire about attitudes and habits that may limit therapy or care.

5. Define the concept of time. Become aware of the patient's and family's perceptions of time and the significance of time frames.

6. Be attentive of interpersonal cues. Determine which ways are most suited for patients and families in terms of how to address the person(s) with whom you are dealing, as well as the symbolic objects or activities that give comfort and security. These recommendations will aid communication between the nurse and the patient or family. The patient–nurse relationship is reciprocal, with the nurse serving as both a learner and a teacher, and the client serving as both a learner and a teacher. Negotiation's purpose is to find a way for people to work together in a collaborative manner to solve an issue or decide on a plan of action. To care for someone, a nurse must first understand who that person is, then understand who the other party is and be able to bridge the gap between them (Anderson, 1987).

Translators' Use

If the client speaks a foreign language, the client's primary language should be used whenever possible. When the nurse does not speak the same language as the patient, it is vital to enlist the help of a translation. Family members, neighbors, and friends, as well as other healthcare personnel and professional interpreters, may act as translators.

III. <u>PREPARING NURSES FOR DIVERSITY CARE</u>

Today, the Philippines is home to a diverse range of cultures, and we are seeing an increase in global migration of people and globalization of nursing practice. The adoption of a culturally informed approach that goes beyond mere language translation and an understanding of the features of other cultures will be critical in providing adequate health care now and in the future.

As caregivers, we must learn to relate to people from varied cultural backgrounds (both patients and colleague healthcare practitioners) and understand the cultural significance of particular health occurrences (Dreher, 1996).

Diversity has the ability to improve our profession by increasing organizational performance, expanding access to treatment, improving patient and staff morale, and increasing labor efficiency (Marquand, 2001).

Increasing minority representation in nursing is an important step in ensuring culturally appropriate nursing care in the twenty-first century. To increase diversity in our ranks, we need to recruit and retain more minority students and staff.

Strengthening multi-cultural perspectives in nursing education programs is another endeavor to break down cultural barriers to health care (Kelley & Fitzsimmons, 2000). Incorporating social ideals that respect varied lifestyles and recognise multicultural and multiracial viewpoints is a key component of innovative nursing education (Sims & Baldwin, 1995). Nurses must not only better grasp the cultural characteristics and attributes of patients and families from various ethnic backgrounds, but also strengthen the connection between nurses and customers from various ethnic backgrounds, according to Dreher (1996). Nurses must be able to establish an atmosphere that encourages patients to express themselves and freely communicate their requirements.

IV. STEREOTYPING: DETERMINING THE SIGNIFICANCE, RISKS, AND SOLUTIONS

"An oversimplified conception, opinion, or belief about some feature of a person or group" is what stereotyping is defined as (Purnell and Paulanka, 1998 p. 490). Stereotyping, according to Woolfolk (1998), is a schema that organizes knowledge or perceptions about a person or group.

Actually, depending on how, where, when, why, and with whom the term is employed, stereotyping can be beneficial or negative. Stereotyping, for example, can be a helpful and acceptable organizing or classifying system if it is founded on logical reasoning and acquired evidence, according to Woolfolk's definition. People can recognize and interpret information using a system of organization and classification, such as "he's Jewish," "she's a Filipino," or "they're Muslims."

Stereotyping, on the other hand, can be harmful if it is used to put someone into a box or an artificial, unfair stance based on oversimplification rather than solid factual support. Negative stereotyping causes people to be disrespected, dehumanized, and denigrated, and it acts as a barrier to equality and fairness.

When stereotypes are coupled with bias or clichés, they get a poor rap.

Stereotyping has a strong emotional component. The positive or bad quality of stereotyping is determined by the languages we use, the attitudes we exhibit, the inferences we draw, and the circumstances in which we use it.

It's simple to generalize someone out of ignorance rather than malice. Nurse educators have a responsibility to stay up to date on the latest research on gender differences, socioeconomic factors, and cultural traditions that influence teaching and learning. Ask yourself the following questions as a nurse educator:

When training clients and families, do I use neutral language?

Do I face bias when other healthcare professionals point it out to me?

Do I ask consumers for the same information regardless of gender, financial background, age, or culture?

Is there any stereotyped wording or idioms in my instructional materials?

Am I a good role model for my coworkers in terms of equality?

Do I handle all clients fairly, respectfully, and with dignity?

Is it true that someone's look influences (raises or lowers) my expectations of their talents or the kind of care I provide?

Do I regularly analyze customers' educational backgrounds, work experiences, personal characteristics, and financial means in order to provide appropriate health education?

Am I familiar enough with other groups' cultural traditions to provide attentive care in our heterogeneous society?

SUMMARY

The impact of gender, socioeconomic level, and cultural attitudes on customers' ability and willingness to learn healthcare measures was investigated in this chapter. The in-depth investigation of these three characteristics can be used to explain various behaviors that have been observed or may be faced in a teaching-learning environment. Although the focus of this chapter was on patients or members of the general public from various ethnic groups with whom nurse educators interact, an understanding of gender differences, socioeconomic influences, and cultural characteristics can also be useful when teaching nursing students or staff from various backgrounds and orientations. The most essential takeaway from this chapter is the importance of being careful not to stereotype or generalize common features of a group to all members of that group. It is acceptable if a nurse does not know much about a culture.

The more significant issue is to inquire about clients' beliefs rather than presuming that they follow the ideals of a certain ethnic group. Nurses can avoid offending the learner this way. The educator must be careful to consider each learner as an individual and determine the amount to which they subscribe to, have beliefs in, or follow practices that may have an impact on learning. Nurses, as professionals, should always seek to improve the quality of care they provide to all individuals, regardless of their gender orientation, ethnicity, creed, nationality, or socioeconomic status (Holtz & Bairan, 1990). Before we can efficiently, confidently, and sensitively offer care to meet the requirements of our socially, cognitively, and culturally diverse clients, nurses need to learn a lot more about how these three elements of gender, socioeconomics, and culture affect the teaching–learning process.

CONTENT EVALUATION

The evaluation after the end of this chapter will be done through a take-home quiz, composed of essay questions, which the students must answer. Citations from other sources must be referenced by way of footnotes. Each paper will go through a plagiarism checker to ensure that none of the answers are copy-pasted. The output shall be submitted through e-mail and shall form part of the student's overall grade.

REVIEW QUESTIONS
1. What are five (5) gender-related differences in cognitive functioning and personality characteristics that affect learning?
2. How does socioeconomic status of individuals influence the teaching-learning process?
3. How can the concept of transcultural nursing be applied to the assessment and teaching of clients from culturally diverse backgrounds?
4. What can the nurse do to avoid cultural stereotyping?
5. Which teaching strategies are most appropriate to meet the needs of individuals from different cultural groups

CHAPTER 8
SPECIAL POPULATIONS

Overview:

This chapter focuses on the nurse's function as an educator in the context of special populations, and it recommends nursing interventions such as teaching self-care strategies to people with a variety of disabilities. The first section of the chapter gives an overview of some of the most frequent disabilities. It focuses on the learning issues that arise in populations with various sorts of deficiencies, as well as the nurse's role as an educator in developing and executing specialized teaching strategies for overcoming communication barriers. It also proposes strategies for nurse educators to accommodate the requirements of disabled patients and their families by incorporating suitable adaptations into their training plans.

Learning Objectives
The student will be able to do the following after finishing this chapter:
1. Recognize the many teaching strategies that work well with students who have learning difficulties.
2. Describe the various physical and mental limitations in order to tailor the teaching-learning strategy appropriately.
3. Improve the teaching-learning process for someone who has difficulty communicating.
4. Talk about how a chronic illness affects people and their families, as well as how it affects the teaching-learning process.

UNIQUE POPULATIONS

Teaching others to be self-sufficient in their life management is an important and difficult duty for nurses in any context and with any population. However, interacting with patients—and, in some cases, nursing staff, nursing students, or hospital personnel—who have altered functional status due to a debilitating illness impacting their physical, cognitive, or sensory capacities makes the teaching-learning process much more difficult. As the nurse's efforts are oriented toward aiding the disabled and their significant others in maintaining existing patterns of life or developing new ones to meet changes in functional capacity, the educational component of nursing practice becomes increasingly important.

I. THE ASSESSMENT ROLE OF THE NURSE AS EDUCATOR

Prior to teaching, clients' needs are always assessed in terms of the nature of their problems, the short- and long-term consequences of their disability, the effectiveness of the coping mechanisms they use, and the type and extent of sensorimotor, cognitive, perceptual, and communication deficits they have. The nurse must identify the depth of the client's disability knowledge, the amount and type of new information required to accomplish a behavior change, and the client's readiness to learn.

When determining a disabled person's readiness to learn, Diehl (1989) suggests asking the following questions:

1. Do the individual and family members show an interest in learning by asking questions or requesting information to solve problems or evaluate their needs?

2. Do you have any learning obstacles, such as limited literacy or eyesight or hearing impairments? Is the client willing and able to use assistive equipment if this is the case?

3. Which learning style is better for digesting information and applying it to self-care tasks for the client?

4. Is there a match between the client's and family's goals?

5. Is the learning environment conducive?

6. Does the client place a high priority on learning new skills and information in order to improve their functional abilities?

7. Does the client associate learning with the possibility of regaining optimal function?

Serving as a mentor to patients and families in coordinating and enabling the diverse services required to assist disabled persons in achieving optimal functioning is a precondition for the nurse's position as a teacher and care giver. As the disabled person's community support system, family and significant others must be invited to participate actively in learning knowledge about assisting with self-care activities for their loved ones from the start.

II. DISABILITIES TYPES

There are two sorts of disabilities that affect millions of people in the United States: mental and physical. These disabilities might have a neurological, physiological, or cognitive foundation, and they can influence thinking processes as well as sensorimotor and neuromuscular functions. Injury, disease, inheritance, or a congenital condition can all cause these problems. The following seven categories have been chosen for discussion to simplify the review of the more common disabilities encountered by nurses in practice: sensory deficits, learning disabilities, developmental disabilities, mental illness, physical disabilities, communication disorders, and chronic illness.

Sensory Deficiencies (A)

1. Hearing Imbalances

- People with impaired hearing, both deaf and hard of hearing, have a total loss or a reduction in sound sensitivity.

- Because there are a variety of ways to communicate with a deaf person, one of the first things you should do is question your client about their communication preferences. Some of the most prevalent options include sign language, written information, lip-reading, and visual aids.

2. Visual Impairments

- A person is determined to be legally blind if vision is 20/200 or less in the better eye with correction or if visual field limits in both eyes are within 20 degrees diameter. Visual impairment is especially common among older persons.

The following are some tips you might find helpful in caring for a blind or visually impaired patient:

1. Secure the services of a low-vision specialist, who can prescribe optical devices such as a magnifying lens (with or without a light), a telescope, a closed-circuit TV, or a pair of sun shields, any of which will enable you to adapt your teaching material to meet the needs of your particular client.

2. Persons who have long-standing blindness have learned to develop a heightened acuity of their other senses of hearing, taste, touch, and smell. Usually, their listening skills are particularly acute, so avoid the tendency to shout. Just because they have impaired vision does not mean they cannot hear you well. Before approaching a visually impaired person, always announce your presence, identify yourself, and explain clearly why you are there and what you are doing.

3. Because their memory and recall also are better than the abilities of most sighted persons, you can use this talent to maximize learning (Babcock & Miller, 1994). When conveying messages, rely on their auditory and tactile senses as a means to help them assimilate information from their environment.

4. When explaining procedures, be as descriptive as possible. Expound on what you are doing, and explain any noises associated with treatments or the use of equipment.

5. Allow the patient to touch, handle, and manipulate equipment. Use the

patient's sense of touch when you are in the process of teaching psychomotor skills as well as when the client is learning to return demonstrate.

6. Arranging things in front of them in a regular clockwise fashion will facilitate learning to perform a task that must be accomplished in an orderly, step-by-step manner (McConnel, 1996).

7. When using printed or handwritten materials, enlarging the print (font size) or handwriting is typically an important first step for those who have diminished sight.

8. Color is a key factor in whether a visually impaired person can distinguish objects. Be sure to assess on which medium your client sees better—black ink on white paper or white ink on black paper. Colors and varying hues of color, other than black and white, are more difficult to discriminate by the older person with vision problems.

9. Proper lighting is of utmost importance in assisting the legally blind person to read the printed word. Regardless of the print size and the color of the type and paper used, if the light is insufficient, the visually impaired person will have a great deal of difficulty reading print or working with objects.

10. Providing contrast is a very helpful technique. For example, using a dark placemat with white dishes or serving black coffee in a white cup will allow persons with visual problems to better see items in front of them.

11. Providing a template (writing guide) for signing their name or writing checks and addressing envelopes is a way to encourage independence.

12. Large-print watches and clocks with either black or white backgrounds are available through the local chapter of the Blind Association.

13. Audiotapes and cassette recorders are very useful tools. Oral instruction can be audiotaped so that blind patients can listen to the information as often as they wish at another time and place. Repetition allows the

opportunity for memorization to reinforce learning.

14. The computer is a popular and useful tool for this population of learners. Although they are costly, some computers have synthetic speech as well as Braille keyboards.

15. If you are assisting the person who is blind to ambulate, always use the "sighted guide" technique; that is, allow the person to grasp your forearm while you walk about one-half step ahead of them.

B. Learning Disabilities

Learning disabilities is "a generic term that refers to a heterogeneous group of disorders manifested by significant difficulties in acquisition and use of listening, speaking, reading, writing, reasoning or mathematical abilities" (Hammill et al., 1981, p. 336). These disorders are intrinsic to the individual and presumed to be due to central nervous dysfunction (Kirk & Kirk, 1983). Individuals with learning disabilities appear normal and have been found to have at least average, if not superior (gifted), intelligence.

The factors that may affect learning in a learning-disabled person are memory, language, motor, and integrative processing disabilities.

The following are some adaptive techniques:

a. Provide information on tape, or give a learner the option of responding to questions orally with a tape recorder.
b. Use hand signs for key words when giving verbal directions.
c. Use hands-on experience or observation.
d. Highlight important information.
e. Use a computer.
f. Capitalize on teachable moments.
g. Use puzzles.
h. Appeal to all senses—auditory, visual, and tactile.
i. Use mnemonics

j. Use a cognitive map

k. Use an active reading strategy such as SQ3R (skim, question, read, rehearse, revise).

C. Developmental Disabilities

A developmental disability, according to the Developmental Disabilities Act of 1978, is a severe chronic condition that begins before the age of 22 and is likely to last indefinitely. It can be brought on by either a mental or physical problem, or a combination of the two.
Self-care, receptive and expressive language learning, mobility, self-direction, capacity for independent living, and economic self-sufficiency are all major life activities that developmentally challenged people have significant limits in.

Managing the treatment of people with developmental impairments is taking up an increasing amount of time in today's healthcare. Nurses must develop sensitivity to family issues and learn to be adaptable in their approaches to satisfy clients' intellectual, emotional, and medical concerns with special needs because developmental disorders are typically identified before infancy and are likely to endure a lifetime.

Consider the client's developmental stage rather than his or her chronological age when organizing an educational intervention. If the kid is unable to communicate vocally, the nurse should record whether the youngster communicates through nonverbal clues such as gestures, signs, or other symbols.

Make sure you don't take over any teaching sessions; instead, allow the child to actively participate and feel accomplished. Assign easy assignments with straightforward instructions. Rather than depending on verbal directions, demonstrate what needs to be done. Only give one instruction at a time. With these patients, an incentive system frequently works quite effectively. Stickers of familiar childhood figures, applied on the child's bed or clothes, might serve as a reminder of a job well done.

Mental Illness (D)

Although there are some special teaching tactics to consider when teaching clients with mental problems, the basic concepts of patient teaching apply.

The client is frequently better equipped to define what he or she needs to learn in non-psychiatric settings. This capacity presupposes that the client is eager to learn. For example, the emotional threat that a person sees as a result of a psychiatric disease may cause a rise in anxiety, which then triggers a cascade of physiological reactions that lowers his or her readiness to learn (Haber et al., 1997).

The first step, like with any other nursing intervention, is to conduct a thorough assessment. In this scenario, it's important to examine the patient's level of anxiety as well as identify whether the client has any cognitive impairment or improper behavior.

The following is a description of three key tactics for teaching persons with mental illness that have proven to be effective (Haber et al., 1997):

1. Teach by using short, basic phrases and repeatedly repeating information—employ mnemonics, record vital information on index cards, and utilize simple images or symbols. Be inventive.

2. Maintain a regular schedule of short and frequent sessions. Instead of a single one-hour session, divide the learning time into four 15-minute sessions.

3. Enlist the assistance of all available resources, including the client and his or her family. Involve them in the process of determining the client's learning styles and the best way to reinforce knowledge. When working with customers, consider using computer-assisted education, videotapes, and role-modeling.

Physical Disabilities are a type of disability that affects a person's ability

1. Injury to the spinal cord

Both the sufferer and the family are affected by a spinal cord injury, which occurs suddenly and without warning. The process of adjustment is challenging and ongoing. During the hospitalization's rehabilitation phase, all interventions are guided by the goal of achieving self-sufficiency. Spinal cord damage causes residual impairment in all aspects of life: physical, social, psychological, vocational, and spiritual.

The nurse must evaluate several frequent difficulties before establishing techniques that help learners to overcome the disability. These problems could be related to or within the learner's ability to participate in the learning process.

When a nurse encounters a person with a spinal cord injury, it is critical that they conduct a thorough assessment of the patient's learning readiness first. The next step is to involve the family and, most significantly, the immediate caretaker, who may or may not be a family member. The client and family will be able to gain and sustain independence with the right assistance and knowledge.

2. Traumatic Brain Injury

Traumatic brain damage can be caused by a fall, a car accident, a gunshot wound, or a hit to the head. The majority of this unique community, which ranges in age from 15 to 24, were formerly healthy and energetic young people. Following a TBI, these individuals frequently have behavioral and personality changes, as well as cognitive impairment.

People who have suffered a severe brain damage are usually treated in three stages:

1. Intensive care (in an intensive care unit)

2. Short-term rehabilitation (in an inpatient brain-injured rehabilitation unit)

3. Post-discharge long-term rehabilitation (at home or in a long-term care facility)

There are numerous obstacles to overcome at each step. The patient is released from the acute care unit once his or her life is ensured and their physical state improves. Someone unfamiliar with traumatic brain injuries may question why a person who appears to be healthy and independent nonetheless requires rehabilitation. As a result, families must be constantly informed about their loved one's prognosis from the start. Family education must be constant and thorough throughout the recovery process, as most residual impairments, with the exception of sensorimotor deficits, are not evident. This population's educational needs are focused on client safety and family coping. Cognitive and behavioral abilities are linked to safety concerns. Families are dealing with a life-altering event that will necessitate continuing assistance and encouragement to care for themselves.

Communication Issues (F)

Humans exchange ideas, sentiments, and wants through communication, which is a universal process. One of the most frustrating feelings is being unable to communicate verbally. One of the first interventions should be speech therapy, and the nurse should incorporate such tactics into the teaching-learning plan. Every attempt must be made to create some kind of contact.

G. Illness that lasts a long time

Unlike acute illnesses, which have a distinct beginning and finish, chronic sickness is a lifelong condition. It can never be fully cured. It necessitates the complete participation of the victims. Physical, psychological, social, economic, and spiritual aspects of life are all impacted. Because managing a chronic illness is a lifelong process, effective learning skills are essential for survival. Individuals with chronic illnesses begin their learning process with rehabilitation at the onset of their handicap. Patients and their families must gain knowledge about the disease and come to an early grasp of its effects on their lives as soon as the problem arises. To deal with the limits and changes in their loved one's lifestyle, families require information and instruction. Feelings of dependence and the desire to be independent are frequently at odds.

The energy and effort required to retain independence can be exhausting, both physically and emotionally. Living with a chronic illness often means losing or changing roles. People's self-esteem may be harmed when they experience role loss (for example, a father who is no longer able to hold his employment).

It's easy to understand how the label of non-compliance may enter the assessment when working with a person with a chronic condition who must maintain a sometimes complex therapeutic regimen (such as a diabetic regimen). The truth is that a chronically ill individual requires more than just teaching—that is, information acquisition. Knowledge does not always lead to the development of new skills needed to deal with difficulties in everyday life. Integration of new knowledge into solutions that provide normalization for clients will make learning more meaningful and, most importantly, helpful. Nurses must remember to encourage patients to stick to their prescribed regimen and to personalize it as needed.

SUMMARY

The shock of any disability, whether it occurs at the beginning of life or toward the end, has a tremendous impact on individuals and their families. At the onset and all through the habilitation or rehabilitation process, the patient and family are met with new information to be learned, as successful habilitation or rehabilitation means acquiring knowledge and applying it to their situation. Inner strength and courage are attributes needed to face each new day, as the effort to live a "normal" life never ends. The physical, social, emotional, and vocational implications of living with a disability necessitate the nurse as an educator to be well prepared to meet any member of this special population right where they are in their struggle to live independently.

REVIEW QUESTIONS

1. What are the major causes of disabilities?
2. Which six (6) questions should be asked by the nurse educator when assessing a disabled person's readiness to learn?
3. What are the seven (7) categories of disabilities?
4. When should the nurse educator enlist the help of a professional interpreter rather than a member of the family when teaching a hearing impaired person?
5. What is the most common obstacle to learning readiness in the special population?

SECTION III
TECHNIQUES AND STRATEGIES FOR TEACHING AND LEARNING

Chapter 9
BEHAVIORAL OBJECTIVES

Overview:

This chapter focuses on the role of behavioral objectives for effective teaching; describes how to write clear and precise behavioral objectives; explores the levels of achievement in the taxonomic hierarchy of cognitive, affective, and psychomotor domains; and outlines the development of teaching plans and learning contracts. All of these elements provide a framework for the successful instruction of the learner.

Learning Outcomes:

After completing this chapter, the student will be able to:

1. Demonstrate the ability to write behavioral objectives accurately and concisely using the three components of condition, performance, and criterion.
2. Distinguish between the three domains of learning.
3. Explain the instructional methods appropriate for teaching in the cognitive, affective, and psychomotor domains.
4. Develop teaching plans that reflect internal consistency between elements.
5. Recognize the role of the nurse educator in formulating objectives for the planning, implementation, and evaluation of teaching and learning.

BEHAVIORAL OBJECTIVES

Whether teaching patients and their families in healthcare settings, training staff nurses in in-service and continuing education programs, or teaching nursing students in academic institutions, the ability to prepare and identify behavioral objectives is a crucial aspect of the educator's position. If data from educational initiatives is to be consistent and measurable, it is critical to understand the procedures for creating and categorizing behavioral objectives for the purpose of specifying learner outcomes.

I. GOAL AND OBJECTIVE CHARACTERISTICS

The terms goal and objective are frequently used interchangeably—albeit incorrectly—despite the fact that there is a significant distinction between the two concepts. Nurse educators must be able to distinguish between the two. The two characteristics that distinguish goals from objectives, and vice versa, are time span and specificity (Haggard, 1989). The goal is what is accomplished at the end of the teaching–learning process. Goals are wide and global in scope, serving as long-term objectives for both the learner and the teacher. Goals are the expected outcomes of learning that can be achieved in a matter of weeks or months. A variety of objectives are subsumed under or incorporated into an overall goal, making them multidimensional. A precise, solitary, unidimensional behavior, on the other hand, is called objective. Short-term objectives should be met at the end of a single teaching session or within a few days after a series of teaching sessions. An aim, according to Mager (1997), is a performance that learners should be able to demonstrate before they are regarded competent. Prior to achieving the goal, objectives must be met. To assess whether the learner has met them, they must be observable and measurable.

A objective can be for a diabetic patient to learn how to manage their diabetes. Specific objectives must be outlined to address behavioral changes such as the need to understand food treatment, insulin administration, exercise regimens, stress management, and glucose monitoring in order to achieve this aim, which has been agreed upon by both the nurse and the patient.

Setting goals and objectives must be a mutual agreement between the teacher and the student if the teaching-learning process is to be successful. The decision-making process must include both parties.

II. BEHAVIORAL OBJECTIVES WRITING

Well-written behavioral objectives provide learners with very clear statements about what is expected of them and help teachers track student progress toward learning outcomes.

The method for establishing short and relevant behavioral objectives, according to Mager (1997), comprises the following three crucial characteristics:

1. Performance: Describes what the learner is anticipated to be able to do or display in order to demonstrate the types of behaviors that the teacher will accept as proof that objectives have been met.

What should a learner be able to accomplish?

2. Condition: Describes the testing scenario or limitations in which the behavior or performance will be observed.

3. Should the student be able to accomplish it under what circumstances?

4. Criterion: The standard, quality level, or amount of performance specified as properly exhibiting mastery; describes how well or with what accuracy the learner must be able to do for the behavior to be regarded acceptable. It refers to the level of proficiency that a student must acquire.

5. How good should the learner be at it?

Mrs. Smith will be able to detect three out of four primary symptoms of low blood sugar (criterion) following a 20-minute teaching session on hypoglycemia (condition)."

III. COMMON OBJECTIVE WRITE-UP MISTAKES

There are a number of frequent traps that both novice and experienced educators might fall into when developing behavioral targets. The following are the most common mistakes made when writing objectives:

a) To state what the instructor, not the student, is supposed to perform.

b) To integrate many required behaviors in a single objective (avoid using compound words and connecting two verbs— for example, the learner will select and prepare).

b) Forgetting to incorporate all three condition, performance, and criterion components.

d) To utilize phrases for performance that can be interpreted in a variety of ways, aren't action-oriented, and are difficult to quantify.

a) To write an unattainable goal based on the learner's current level of skill.

f) Writing objectives that have nothing to do with the stated goal.

a) To clog up an objective by including irrelevant information.

h) To be too broad in order to avoid explicitly stating the desired consequence

I. **TAXONOMY OF OBJECTIVES ACCORDING TO LEARNING DOMAINS**

A taxonomy is a system for classifying objects based on their relationships with one another. The Taxonomy of Educational Objectives was established by Bloom et al. (1956) and Knathwohl and associates (1964) as a tool for methodically identifying behavioral objectives. This taxonomy is organized into three basic categories or domains: cognitive, emotional, and psychomotor. It has been generally regarded as a standard guide for planning and analyzing learning.

The Cognitive Domain (A).

The "thinking" domain is part of the cognitive domain. In this domain, learning refers to the learner's intellectual abilities, mental capacities, and thinking processes, as well as the acquisition of information. The domain's objectives are separated into six levels, each of which specifies cognitive processes ranging from the simple (knowledge) to the more sophisticated (perception) (evaluation),

Cognitive Behavior Levels

1. Knowledge: the learner's ability to memorize, recall, define, recognize, or identify specific information offered during education, such as facts, rules, principles, conditions, and words.

Choose, circle, define, identify, label, list, match, name, outline, recall, report, choose, state are just a few examples.

2. Comprehension: the learner's ability to show that he or she understands or appreciates what is being communicated by translating it into a different form or recognizing it in a translated form, such as grasping an idea by defining or summarizing it in his or her own words (knowledge is a prerequisite behavior).

Describe, discuss, differentiate, estimate, explain, generalize, give an example, find, recognize, and so on.

3. Application: the learner's capacity to apply concepts, principles, abstractions, or theories in specific and concrete situations, such as calculating, writing, reading, or operating machinery (knowledge and comprehension are prerequisite behaviors).

Apply, demonstrate, illustrate, implement, interpret, modify, order, revise, solve, and use are some examples of verbs.

4. Analysis: the learner's ability to recognize and structure information by dissecting it into its constituent elements and describing the relationships between them (knowledge, comprehension, and application are prerequisite behaviors).

Organize, calculate, classify, compare, conclude, contrast, determine, discriminate, etc.

5. Synthesis: the learner's capacity to combine parts and elements together to form a coherent whole by creating a one-of-a-kind result that is written, spoken, graphical, and so on (knowledge, comprehension, application, and analysis are prerequisite behaviors).

Examples include categorize, combine, compile, correlate, design, devise, produce, integrate, reorganize, revise, and summarize.

6. Evaluation: the learner's capacity to assess the worth of anything, such as an essay, a design, or an activity, using suitable standards or criteria (knowledge, comprehension, application, analysis, and synthesis are prerequisite behaviors).

7. Examine, evaluate, conclude, criticize, debate, defend, judge, and justify

Affective Domain (B)

The emotional domain is commonly referred to as the "feeling" domain. Internalization or commitment to sentiments represented as emotions, interests, attitudes, values, and appreciations is a key component of learning in this domain. The cognitive domain is separated into categories that indicate the depth of a person's emotional responses to activities, whereas the affective domain is divided into categories that specify the degree of a person's emotional responses to tasks (Reilly & Oerman, 1990).

Although nurse educators appreciate the importance of individuals learning in the emotive domain, categories like attitudes, beliefs, and values can only be inferred from words and actions (Maier-Lorentz, 1999). Competence in the emotive domain is required of staff nurses in order to intervene with clients in a humanistic and compassionate manner.

The terms beliefs, attitudes, and values are defined by Reilly and Oermann (1990). Values are operational beliefs that guide actions and ways of living. Beliefs are what an individual perceives as reality; attitudes are feelings towards an object, person, or event; and values are operational beliefs that guide actions and ways of living.

Affective Behavior Levels

1. Receiving: the learner's ability to demonstrate knowledge of an idea or truth, as well as awareness of a situation or event in the surroundings. This level denotes a willingness to pay attention to or focus on data or receive a stimulus selectively.

Accept, admit, ask, attend, focus, listen, observe, pay attention, accept, acknowledge, admit, confess, admit, admit, admit, admit, admit, admit, admit, admit, admit,

2. Responding: the learner's ability to respond to an event, at first obediently, then willingly and happily. This stage denotes a transition from denial to voluntary acceptance, which may result in sentiments of pleasure or happiness as a result of a new experience (receiving is a prerequisite behavior).

For example, agree, answer, conform, discuss, express, participate, recollect, relate, report, demonstrate willingness, try, and verbalize.

3. Valuing: the learner's ability to regard or embrace the worth of a theory, idea, or event, displaying sufficient commitment or preference to be connected with a valuable experience. There is a clear willingness and desire to act to promote that value at this level (receiving and responding are prerequisite behaviors).

Assert, assist, attempt, pick, finish, disagree, follow, aid, initiate, join, propose, volunteer

4. Organization: the learner's ability to organize, classify, and prioritize values by incorporating a new value into a larger set of values, determining value interrelationships, and harmoniously establishing some values as dominant and ubiquitous (receiving, responding, and valuing are prerequisite behaviors).

Adhere, alter, arrange, combine, defend, explain, express, generalize, integrate, and resolve are just a few examples.

5. Characterization: the learner's ability to integrate values into a larger philosophy or worldview, demonstrating solid commitment and consistency in reactions to values by generalizing specific experiences into a value system or attitude cluster (receiving, responding, valuing, and organization are prerequisite behaviors).

Assert, commit, differentiate, display, influence, propose, qualify, solve, and verify are some examples of verbs.

Domain of Psychomotor

The "skills" domain refers to the psychomotor domain. Learning in this domain include developing fine and gross motor skills, as well as increasing the complexity of neuromuscular coordination, in order to perform bodily movements like walking, handwriting, manipulating equipment, or performing a procedure. According to Reilly and Oermann (1990), "psychomotor skill learning is a complex process requiring significantly more understanding than implied by the simple mechanistic behavioral approach" (p. 81).

Psychomotor Behavior Levels

1. Perception: the client's ability to demonstrate sensory awareness of things or cues linked with a task to be completed. Cues pertinent to the circumstance are recognized, symbolically translated, and chosen to drive action, obtain understanding, and receive feedback. This level entails reading instructions or witnessing a process while paying close attention to the steps or strategies involved.

Attend, choose, describe, detect, differentiate, distinguish, identify, isolate, perceive, relate, choose, and separate are some examples of words.

2. Set: the learner's ability to show readiness to perform a specific action, such as following directions, through expressions of willingness, sensory attending, or body language that is conducive to performing a motor act (perception is a prerequisite behavior).

Attempt, begin, develop, display, position, prepare, continue, reach, reply, show, start, try are some examples.

3. Guided response: the learner's ability to expend effort through overt actions while being guided by an instructor to repeat an observed behavior while being mindful of effort. Imitating can be done tentatively, but with the right guidance and coaching, it can be done successfully (perception and set are prerequisite behaviors).

4. Mechanism: the learner's ability to confidently perform steps of a desired skill over and over again, indicating mastery to the point where some or all aspects of the process become habitual. The steps are seamlessly integrated into a meaningful whole and carried out with little conscious effort (perception, set, and guided response are prerequisite behaviors).

5. Complex overt response: the learner's ability to automatically perform a complex motor act with independence and a high level of skill, without hesitation and with minimal time and energy expenditure; the ability to perform an entire sequence of a complex behavior without the need to pay attention to details (perception, set, guided response, and mechanism are prerequisite behaviors).

8. Guided response, mechanism, and complex overt response: align, arrange, attach, build, change, choose, clean, compile, complete, construct, demonstrate, discriminate, dismantle, dissect, examine, find, grasp, hold, insert, lift, locate, maintain, manipulate, measure, mix, open, operate, organize, perform, pour, practice, reassemble, remove, repair, replace, shake, suction

6. Adaptation: the learner's ability to change or adjust a motor process to suit the individual or different contexts, suggesting mastery of highly developed motions that may be used in a range of situations (perception, set, guided response, mechanism, and complex overt response are prerequisite behaviors).

Adapt, change, convert, correct, rearrange, reorganize, replace, revise, shift, substitute, and switch are just a few examples.

7. Origination: ability of the learner to create new motor acts, such as novel ways of manipulating objects or materials, as a result of an understanding of a skill and developed ability to perform skills (perception, set, guided response, mechanism, complex overt response, and adaptation are prerequisite behaviors).

Ex. arrange, combine, compose, construct, create, design, exchange, reformulate

II. **DEVELOPMENT OF TEACHING PLANS**

After mutually agreed-upon goals and objectives have been written, it should be clear what the learner is to learn and what the teacher is to teach. Predetermined goals and objectives serve as a basis for developing a *teaching plan*.

The three major reasons for constructing teaching plans are:

1. To force the teacher to examine the relationship among the steps of the teaching process to ensure a logical approach to teaching, which can serve as a map for organizing and keeping instruction on target.

2. To communicate in writing and in an outline format exactly what is being taught, how it is being taught and evaluated, and the time allotted for accomplishment of the behavioral objectives. As such, not only is the learner aware of and can follow the action plan, but, just as importantly, other healthcare team members are informed and can contribute to the teaching effort with a consistent approach.

3. To legally document that an individual plan for each learner is in place and is being properly implemented.

    A complete teaching plan consists of eight basic parts (Ryan & Marinelli, 1990):

    1) The purpose
    2) A statement of the overall goal
    3) A list of objectives (and sub-objectives, if necessary)
    4) An outline of the related content

5) The instructional method(s) used for teaching the related content
6) The time allotted for the teaching of each objective
7) The instructional resources (materials/tools) needed
8) The method(s) used to evaluate learning

The overall design of the teaching plan must match whatever domain(s) of learning have been selected, as identified below:

Table 3. Teaching Design for each Domain

Domain	Teaching Design
Cognitive	Topic-centered
Affective	Feeling-centered
Psychomotor	Performance-centered

III. <u>USE OF LEARNING CONTRACTS</u>

The concept of *learning contracts* is a relatively new but increasingly popular approach to teaching and learning that can be implemented with any audience of learners—patients and their families, nursing staff, or nursing students.

In the strictest sense, a contract is a formal legal agreement governing the terms of a transaction over a specified period of time between two or more parties (O'Reilly, 1994). In education, a learning contract is defined as a written (formal) or verbal (informal) agreement between the teacher and the learner that delineates specific teaching and learning activities that are to occur within a certain time frame.

A learning contract is a mutually negotiated agreement, usually in the form of a written document drawn up by the teacher and the learner, that specifies what the learner will learn, how learning will be achieved and within what time allotment, and the criteria for measuring the success of the venture (Keyzer, 1986; McAllister, 1996).

Four Major Components of the Learning Contract (Wallace & Mundie, 1987):

1) *Content*—specifies the precise behavioral objectives to be achieved. Objectives must clearly state the desired outcomes of learning activities. Negotiation between the educator and the learner determines the content, level, and sequencing of objectives according to learner needs, abilities, and readiness.

2) *Performance expectations*—specify the conditions under which learning activities will be facilitated, such as instructional strategies and resources.

3) *Evaluation*—specifies the criteria used to evaluate achievement of objectives, such as skills checklists, care standards or protocols, and agency policies and procedures of care that identify the levels of competency expected of the learner.

4) *Time frame*—specifies the length of time needed for successful completion of the objectives. The target date for completion should reflect a reasonable period in which to achieve expected outcomes depending on the learner's abilities and circumstances.

Steps to Implement the Learning Contract:

Step 1: *Determine specific learning objectives.* Encourage the learner to identify his or her learning needs and what the learner wants to be able to do within an allotted time frame.

Step 2: *Review the contracting process.* It is vital that learners have a complete understanding of what contract learning is all about as well as their role in the process. Because learning contracts have not been widely used until recently, most people are unfamiliar with this teaching-learning strategy.

Step 3: *Identify the learning resources.* Introduce the learner to instructional resources available, such as self-study materials and audiovisual tools.

Step 4: *Assess the learner's competency level and learning needs.* The entire process of negotiation of a contract is based on the learner's current abilities and learning needs. The educator initiates the assessment of the learner and collects data primarily through interview, observation, and pretesting to formulate objectives.

Step 5: *Define roles.* Before planning learning experiences and negotiating a contract, the roles of the learner and the educator must be clearly established regarding expectations of each.

Step 6: *Plan the learning experiences.* Determine the content, learning resources to be used, the skills that must be demonstrated, and the amount of time to pursue learning through assisted or self-study to meet the predetermined objectives.

Step 7: *Negotiate the time frame.* Based on appropriate sequencing of behaviors, from simplest to most complex, establish a target date for completion of each objective.

Step 8: *Implement the learning experience.* Take into consideration individual variations in the level of ability to do self-directed study and any other variables that may play a factor in the completion of the specified learning activities. For patients, progress in learning may be influenced by changes in their health status. For staff nurses, the constant pressures of providing patient care services may place constraints on the time available for educational activities. For any learner, the education process is influenced by readiness to learn and how well the information to be learned is organized and communicated.

Step 9: *Renegotiate.* The type and level of complexity of behavioral objectives and the target dates set forth for accomplishing these objectives may be renegotiated at any point along the learning experience continuum to meet the learner's needs. Adults may change their notions about what they want to learn, how they want to learn it, and how long it will take to achieve objectives, so they should be encouraged to revise their contract as it is being carried out.

Step 10. *Evaluate.* Periodic (formative) and final (summative) evaluation of the learner's progress and the actual learning experience itself is a shared responsibility between the learner and the educator. Pre-established performance criteria, agreed on prior to the initiation of the learning process, serve as the means to ascertain achievement of outcomes based on predetermined and pre-negotiated behavioral objectives.

Step 11: *Document.* Evidence of achievement of learning objectives is determined jointly by the learner and the educator (and preceptors if used for nursing staff and students). When an objective is satisfactorily met according to written performance expectations, each party cosigns the date completed in the appropriate column.

SUMMARY

The major portion of this chapter focused on differentiating goals from objectives, preparing accurate and concise objectives, classifying objectives according to the three domains of learning, and teaching cognitive, affective, and psychomotor skills using appropriate instructional interventions. The writing of behavioral objectives as to type and complexity is fundamental to the education process. Goals and objectives guide the educator in the planning, implementation, and evaluation of teaching and learning. Assessment of the learner is a prerequisite to formulating objectives. Objectives setting must be a partnership effort by the learner and the educator for any learning experience to be successful and rewarding in achieving expected outcomes. This chapter also outlined the development of teaching plans and learning contracts. Teaching plans provide the blueprint for organizing and presenting information in a coherent manner. Above all else, a teaching plan must reflect internal consistency of its parts. Learning contracts are an innovative and unique alternative to structuring a learning experience based on adult learning principles. Contracts are designed to provide for self-directed study, thereby encouraging active involvement and accountability on the part of the learner.

REVIEW QUESTIONS

1. What is the difference between the terms *educational* or *instructional objectives*?
2. What two (2) major factors distinguish goals and objectives from one another?
3. What is the definition of the terms *goal* and *objective*?
4. What are the three (3) major characteristics that should be included in every written behavioral objective?
5. What eight (8) mistakes are commonly made when writing behavioral objectives?
6. What are the three (3) domains of learning?
7. Why is it important for the educator to remember to keep psychomotor skill instruction separate from the cognitive and affective components of skill development?
8. What are the eight (8) basic components of a teaching plan?
9. Why are learning contracts an increasingly popular approach to teaching and learning?
10. What are the four (4) major components of a learning contract?

CHAPTER 10
INSTRUCTIONAL METHODS

Overview:

This chapter will review the types of instructional methods available and consider how to choose and use them efficiently and effectively. It will also identify the strengths and limitations of each method, the variables influencing the selection of various techniques, and ways to evaluate the methods used to improve the delivery of instruction. Throughout, examples will be drawn from a variety of learners, such as the person in a wellness program trying to stop smoking, the patient learning how to self-manage his or her diabetes, and the staff nurse learning to coordinate a cardiac arrest, because the nurse is expected to teach a variety of learners in a variety of settings.

Learning Outcomes

After completing this chapter, the student will be able to:

1. Explain the various types of instructional methods.
2. Describe how to use each method effectively.
3. Identify the strengths and limitations of each method.
4. Discuss the variables that influence the selection of a method.
5. Recognize strategies to enhance teaching effectiveness.

INSTRUCTIONAL METHODS

Instructional strategy is the overall plan for a learning experience. It involves the use of one or several methods of teaching, and it encompasses both the content and the process that will be used to achieve the desired outcomes of instruction (Rothwell & Kazanas, 1992).

Instructional methods are the techniques or approaches the teacher uses to bring the learner into contact with the content to be learned.

Methods are a way, an approach, or a process to communicate information. Some examples of methods are lecture, group discussion, one-to-one instruction, demonstration and return demonstration, gaming, simulation, role-playing, role modeling, self-instruction chapters, computer-assisted instruction, and distance learning techniques

Instructional materials or *tools* are the actual vehicles by which information is shared with the learner. Books, videos, and posters are examples of materials and tools.

I. <u>TYPES OF INSTRUCTIONAL METHODS</u>

Instructional methods can be categorized in many ways. The rationale for the classification reflects whether the learner's role is active or passive, the technique is student- or instructor-centered, or the focus is on content versus process knowledge.

A. Traditional Methods

The traditional methods tend to have more teacher input and control during encounters with the learner than do the less traditional formats. The traditional methods include lecture, group discussion, one-to-one instruction, demonstration, and return demonstration.

1) **Lecture** can be defined as a highly structured method by which the teacher verbally transmits information directly to groups of learners for the purpose

of instruction. It is one of the oldest and most often used methods.

- Lecture format allows for only minimal exchange between the teacher and the learner, but it can be an effective method of teaching in the lower-level cognitive domain to impart content knowledge. Lecture is an efficient, cost-effective method for getting large amounts of information across to a large number of people all at the same time as well as within a relatively reasonable time frame.

- With respect to its limitations, the lecture method is ineffective in influencing affective and psychomotor behaviors. It does not provide for much stimulation of learners, and there is little opportunity for learner involvement. Rather, learners are passive recipients of the information being presented. The focus, instead, is very instructor-centered, and thus the most active participant is frequently the most knowledgeable one—the teacher.

2) **Group discussion** is a method of teaching whereby learners get together to exchange information, feelings, and opinions with one another and with the teacher. Discussion is one of the most commonly employed instructional techniques. The activity is learner-centered and subject-centered.

- The major advantage of group discussion is that it stimulates learners to think about issues and problems and to exchange their own experiences, thereby making learning more active.

3) **One-to-one instruction** - the teacher delivers individual instruction designed specifically for a particular learner.

- It is an opportunity to communicate ideas and feelings primarily through oral exchange, although nonverbal messages can be conveyed as well.

4) **Demonstration and Return**

- *Demonstration* is a method by which the learner is shown by the teacher how to perform a particular skill.
- *Return demonstration* is the method by which the learner attempts to

perform the skill with cues from the teacher as needed.
- ➢ These two methods require different abilities by both the teacher and the learner. Each is effective in teaching psychomotor domain skills. Both may also enhance cognitive and affective learning—for example, when helping someone develop interactive skills to be used in crisis intervention or assertiveness training.

B. Nontraditional Methods

In the nontraditional approaches, teachers act more as designers and facilitators than as verbal presenters and givers of information. Nontraditional methods include gaming, simulation, role-playing, role-modeling, self-instruction activities, computer-assisted instruction, and distance learning.

1) **Gaming** is an instructional method requiring the learner to participate in a competitive activity with preset rules. These activities do not have to reflect reality, but they are designed to accomplish educational objectives.
    - ➢ The goal is for the learners to win a game by applying knowledge and rehearsing skills previously learned.
    - ➢ It promotes retention of information by stimulating learner enthusiasm and increasing learner involvement.
    - ➢ Gaming is fun with a purpose. This method adds variety to the learning experience and is excellent for dull or repetitious content that requires periodic review.

2) **Role-playing** is a method by which learners participate in an unrehearsed dramatization. They are asked to play assigned parts of a character as they think the character would act in reality.

    - ➢ This method is a technique to arouse feelings and elicit emotional responses in the learner. It is used primarily to achieve behavioral objectives in the affective domain.

    - ➢ Role-playing differs from simulation, where learners rehearse behaviors or roles that they will need to master and apply in real life. For example, the patients in a diabetes self-management education program will need to practice behaviors such as selecting foods from a restaurant menu and setting their insulin pumps for the correct bolus of insulin because these are self-management skills they are trying to master. In role-playing, on the other hand, the learner is not mastering a role with plans to use it but rather to develop understanding of other people. The nurse attending an education program, for instance, may wear an insulin pump containing saline and select the appropriate foods to "see how it feels" to have to be aware of these issues rather than for the purpose of mastering the techniques.

3) **Role-Modeling** - Learning from *role-modeling* is called identification and emanates from socialization theories that explain how people acquire new behaviors and social roles.
    - Nurse educators have many opportunities to demonstrate behaviors and attitudes they would like to instill in learners, whether patients, family members, nursing staff, or students.

4) **Self-instruction Activities** is a method the teacher uses to provide or design instructional activities that guide the learner in independently achieving the objectives of learning. Each self-study chapter usually focuses on one topic, and the hallmark of this format is independent study.
    - The self-instruction method is effective for learning in the cognitive and psychomotor domains, where the goal is to master information and apply it to practice.

5) **Computer-assisted instruction** (CAI) is an individualized method of self-study using computers to deliver an educational activity.
    - CAI allows learners to proceed at their own pace with immediate and continuous feedback on their progress as they respond to a software program.

6) **Distance learning** is a telecommunications approach to instruction using video technology to transmit live or taped messages directly from the instructor to the viewer.
    - It is becoming more popular as an instructional technique for staff development, continuing education programs, and student learning in academic settings. Distance learning is made possible by network technology

II. SELECTION OF INSTRUCTIONAL METHODS

The process of selecting an instructional method requires a prior determination of the behavioral objectives to be accomplished and an assessment of the learners who will be involved in achieving the objectives.

Consideration must be given to available resources such as time, money, space, and materials to support learning activities. The teacher is also an important variable in the selection and effectiveness of a method.

III. EVALUATION OF INSTRUCTIONAL METHODS

An important aspect of evaluating any instructional program is to assess the effectiveness of the method. Was the choice selected as effective, efficient, and appropriate as possible?

There are five major questions to ask yourself that will help you to decide which method to choose or if the method selected should be revised or rejected:

1. *Does the method help the learners to achieve the stated objectives?* This question is the most important criterion for evaluation—if the method does not accomplish the objectives, then all the other criteria are unimportant. Will the method expose learners to the necessary information and training to learn the desired behaviors?

2. *Is the learning activity accessible to the learners you have targeted?* Accessibility includes when information is presented, the location and setting in which teaching takes place, and the availability of resources and equipment to deliver your message. Patients and family members need programs to be offered at suitable times and accessible locations. For example, childbirth preparation classes scheduled during the daytime hours would likely not be convenient for expectant couples who are working.

3. *Is the method efficient given the time, energy, and resources available in relation to the number of learners you are trying to reach?* To teach large numbers of learners, you will have to choose a method that can accommodate groups, such as lecture, discussion sessions, or role-playing,

or a method that can reach many individuals at one time, such as the use of various self-instructional formats or CAI.

4. *To what extent does the method allow for active participation to accommodate the needs, abilities, and style of the learner?* Active participation has been well documented as a way to increase interest in learning and the retention of information.

5. *Is the method cost-effective?* It is vital to examine the cost of educational programs to determine whether similar outcomes might be achieved by using less costly methodologies.

IV. <u>INCREASING EFFECTIVENESS OF TEACHING</u>

Excellent teachers have one thing in common - a passion to keep improving their abilities. One does not "arrive" at being an expert teacher. The drive toward excellence is an ongoing process that continues throughout the teacher's entire professional life. What constitutes creative teaching? What personal attributes does the creative teacher possess?

Creative Techniques to Enhance the Effectiveness of Verbal Presentations

- ✓ *Present information enthusiastically.* The teacher who comes across as invested in the material excites the learner to identify with the subject at hand. No matter how well a lesson is planned or how clearly it is presented, if it is delivered in a dry and dull monotone, it will likely fall on deaf ears

- ✓ *Include humor.* Many creative teachers use humor as a technique to grab, arouse, and maintain the attention of the learner. Appropriate humor can help establish a rapport with learners by humanizing the teacher.

- ✓ *Exhibit risk-taking behavior.* Creative teachers are willing to develop exercises in which many variables can lead to any number of possible outcomes. They use this technique to encourage learners to reach their own conclusions about controversial issues

- ✓ *Deliver material dramatically.* Creative teachers seek ways to engage the learner emotionally by using surprise, controlled tension, or ploys. The teacher uses strategies that connect the educational material directly to the learner's life experiences to make information more understandable and relevant.

- ✓ *Choose problem-solving activities.* Whether the learners are staff members or patients, the creative teacher recognizes that learners need to be immersed in activities to help them develop problem-solving skills.

- ✓ *Serve as a role model.* The creative teacher constantly seeks new information by keeping abreast of current research, theories, and issues in clinical practice for application relevant to the teaching situation.

- ✓ *Use anecdotes and examples.* The creative teacher uses stories, tales, and examples of incidences and episodes to illustrate points.

- ✓ *Use technology.* Creative teachers use technology to broaden and add variety to the opportunities for teaching and learning. They continue to increase their own skills by taking advantage of the advances in technology to introduce and coach others in new ways of learning.

SUMMARY

This chapter has presented all of the major traditional and nontraditional methods of instruction. Emphasis was given to the importance of considering the learner characteristics, behavioral objectives, teacher characteristics, and available resources prior to selecting or designing any of the vast arrays of methods at the teacher's disposal. Guidelines were put forth to assist nurse educators in planning and to develop their own instructional activities. In addition, the major questions to be considered when evaluating the effectiveness of instructional methods were assessed in detail. Lastly, but equally as important as selecting the right method, were the strategies a creative teacher uses and the general principles all teachers should use to communicate with learners effectively. What must be stressed are the inherent qualities of each method and the fact that no one method is better than another. Nurses in the role of educators are urged to take an eclectic approach to teach by avoiding reliance on any one particular method and by using a combination of teaching methods to accomplish the objectives for learning while at the same time meeting the different needs and styles of every learner.

REVIEW QUESTIONS

1. How is the term *instructional method* defined?
2. Which instructional methods are considered to be traditional and which are considered to be nontraditional?
3. Which instructional methods are best for learning cognitive skills? Psychomotor skills? Affective skills?
4. What are the six (6) variables that influence the selection of any method of instruction?
5. What major questions should you ask yourself when evaluating the effectiveness of any instructional method?
6. What are the techniques that creative teachers use to enhance the effectiveness of teaching?
7. Are teachers born or made? Explain
8. What quality do all expert teachers have in common?

CHAPTER 11
INSTRUCTIONAL MATERIALS

Overview:

This chapter provides an overview of the process for selecting, developing, using, and evaluating instructional materials. A systematic approach is taken to examine various types of instructional media with an eye to matching their use to the particular characteristics of learners and specific topics and situations. This chapter is intended to inform nurse educators about various media options and allow them to make informed choices regarding appropriate instructional materials that fit the learner, that will accomplish the learning task, and that will affect the motivation of the learner.

Learning Outcomes
After completing this chapter, the student will be able to:

1. Differentiate between instructional materials and methods of instruction.
2. Identify the three major variables (learner, task, and media characteristics) to be considered when selecting, developing, and evaluating instructional materials.
3. Describe guidelines for development of printed materials.
4. Analyze the advantages and disadvantages specific to each type of instructional medium.
5. Evaluate the type of media suitable for use depending on the characteristics of the audience, seating, preference, resources available, nature of the subject, and characteristics of the learner, such as age, literacy level, and sensory deficits.

INSTRUCTIONAL MATERIALS

Whereas *instructional methods* are the approaches or processes used for instructor–client communications, *instructional materials* are the resources and tools used as vehicles to help communicate the information.

Instructional materials are tangible substances and real objects that provide the audio and/or visual component necessary for learning. Many of them can be manipulated. They stimulate a learner's senses and may have the power to arouse emotions. They help the teacher make sense of abstractions and simplify complex messages (Babcock & Miller, 1994). [1]

I. **CHOOSING INSTRUCTIONAL MATERIALS**

Many important variables must be considered when choosing instructional materials. The role of the nurse educator goes beyond the dispensing of information only; it also involves skill in designing and planning for instruction. Learning can be made more enjoyable for both the learner and the teacher if the educator knows what instructional materials are available and how to select and use them to enhance the teaching-learning experience. [2]

Making appropriate choices of instructional materials depends on a broad understanding of three major variables: LMAT: **L**earner, **M**edia, **a**nd **T**ask.

1. *Characteristics of the learner* (L): As variables in the learner are known to influence learning, it is important to "know your audience" to choose media that best suits their needs. You must consider the learners' perceptual, physical, reading, motivational levels (locus of control), developmental stages, and learning styles.

2. *Characteristics of the media* (M): The nurse educator has the opportunity to choose from a wide variety of media, print and non-print, to enhance methods of instruction. Non-print media include the full range of audio and visual possibilities. The tools selected are the form through which the information will be communicated. No single medium is most effective. Therefore, the educator must be flexible, sometimes combining a

multimedia approach. [3]

3. *Characteristics of the task* (T): Task characteristics are defined by predetermined behavioral objectives. The task to be accomplished depends on the identification of the learning domain and the complexity of behavior required by the task.

II. **THE THREE MAJOR COMPONENTS OF INSTRUCTIONAL MATERIALS**

Whatever instructional method is used, decisions will also have to be made regarding the media necessary to help communicate information. The delivery system (Weston & Cranston, 1986), content, and presentation (Frantz, 1980) are the three major components of media that should be kept in mind when evaluating print and non-print materials for potential instruction. [4]

A. **Delivery System** - The *delivery system* is both the physical form of the materials and the hardware used to present the materials. For instance, a person is the delivery system for a lecture. This lecture might be embellished through other delivery systems, such as the use of overhead transparencies or slides (physical form), and a projector (hardware). Videotapes (physical form) in conjunction with VCRs (hardware) and computer programs (physical form) in conjunction with the computer (hardware) are other examples. [4]

➢ The delivery system is independent of the content of the message. The choice of the delivery system is influenced by the size of the intended audience, the pacing or flexibility needed for delivery, and the sensory aspects most suitable to the audience.

B. **Content** - The content, or message, is the actual information that is communicated to the learner, which might be on any topic from sexuality to educational psychology. When selecting media, the nurse educator must consider several aspects:

✓ Is the information presented accurately?
✓ Is the medium chosen appropriate to convey particular content?

- ✓ Is the readability of the materials appropriate for the audience to accomplish a given task?

C. Presentation

Frantz (1980) describes presentation as those variables that affect the way in which the content or message to be learned is delivered. Weston and Cranston (1986) state that the form of the message is the most important consideration for selecting or developing instructional materials, a consideration that is frequently ignored. They describe the form of the message as occurring along a continuum from concrete (real objects) to abstract (symbols). [5]

III. <u>TYPES OF INSTRUCTIONAL MATERIALS</u>

A. **Written Materials** - Handouts, leaflets, books, pamphlets, brochures, and instruction sheets are the most widely employed and most accessible type of media used for teaching.

- ➢ The use of printed materials offers some distinct advantages. The greatest virtue of written materials is that they are available to the learner as a reference for information when the nurse educator is not immediately present to answer questions or clarify information.

B. **Demonstration Materials** - Demonstration materials include many types of non-print media, such as models and real equipment, as well as displays, such as posters, diagrams, illustrations, charts, bulletin boards, flannel boards, flip charts, chalkboards, photographs, and drawings. [6]

- ➢ All represent unique ways of communicating messages to the learner. These aids primarily stimulate the visual senses but can combine the sense of sight with touch and sometimes even smell and taste.

C. **Audiovisual Materials** - support and enrich the educational process by stimulating the learner's visual and auditory senses, adding variety to the teaching-learning experience, and instilling visual memories, which have been found to be more permanent than auditory memories (de Tornyay &

Thompson, 1987).

IV. EVALUATION CRITERIA FOR SELECTING MATERIALS

Choosing the right tools for patient education calls for judgment on the nurse educator, who must consider the *learner*, the *task*, and the *media* available to help achieve learning objectives. Decisions may need to be made on an individual basis or for large groups, depending on the size and characteristics of the audience. There may be multiple objectives. The educator must consider the media available in general, but different objectives may best be reached with different teaching materials.

Table 4. Effectiveness of teaching tools and methods

Mode of Learning	Retention	Media	Methods
Reading	Learners retain 10% of what they read.	Leaflets, books, brochures, flip charts, chalkboards, instruction sheets	Self-instruction
Hearing	Learners retain 20% of what they hear.	Audiotapes, telephones	Lectures, discussion
Watching	Learners retain 30% of what they see.	Silent films, displays, photos, pictures, posters, cartoons, drawings	Demonstration, self-instruction
Watching and hearing	Learners retain 50% of what they see and hear.	Movies (films), TV, videotapes, slides, overheads, models	Lecture or demonstration
Watching and speaking	Learners retain 70% of what they see and talk about.	Audiovisual media	Group discussion, 1:1 verbal interactions, demonstrations
Speaking and doing	Learners retain 90% of what they talk about and do.	Interactive media	Demonstration, return demonstration, gaming, role-playing

SUMMARY

This chapter discussed the major categories of instructional materials and answered questions about how to select media from a range of possible options and how to evaluate their effectiveness. Nurse educators are expected to make these choices every day, whether it is to meet the needs of an individual learner or to design a large educational program to satisfy a broader, more diverse group. In this chapter, the importance of considering characteristics of the learner, the media, and the task when choosing instructional materials was emphasized. The supplemental nature of teaching materials was also stressed and the need to keep the teaching objectives and behavioral objectives in focus when selecting these materials as adjuncts to instruction.

CONTENT EVALUATION

The evaluation after the end of this chapter will be done through a take-home quiz, which the students must answer. Citations from other sources must be referenced by way of footnotes. Each paper will go through a plagiarism checker to ensure that none of the answers are copy-pasted. The output shall be submitted through e-mail and shall form part of the student's overall grade.

REVIEW QUESTIONS

1. How do instructional materials differ from instructional methods?
2. What are the three (3) major variables to consider when selecting, developing, and evaluating instructional materials?
3. What are the major advantages and disadvantages of computer learning resources?
4. Why is the statement true that instructional materials should not be selected before behavioral objectives are determined?
5. Which two (2) modes of learning are most effective for the retention of information? Why?

CHAPTER 12
TECHNOLOGY IN EDUCATION

Overview:

This chapter is designed as an introduction to the use of technology in education. Because nurses provide both healthcare and professional education, it will address technology-based resources and strategies appropriate for use with clients and with nurses and other healthcare professionals. The chapter will provide a basic overview of the technology involved and implications for the educator and the learner. Chapter 11 discusses the use of audiovisual materials in the classroom. Hence, this chapter will focus primarily on the Internet, the World Wide Web, and computer-based hardware and software applications that can be used to enhance learning with students in the classroom as well as with learners at a distance. [1]

Learning Outcomes:
After completing this chapter, the student will be able to:

1. Describe changes in education that have occurred as a result of Information Age technology.
2. Identify ways in which the resources of the Internet and World Wide Web could be incorporated into healthcare education.
3. Describe the role of the nurse educator in using technology in client and

staff education.
4. Recognize the issues related to the use of technology
5. Discuss the effects that technology has had on professional education for nurses. [2]

TECHNOLOGY IN EDUCATION

The birth of the Internet and the World Wide Web, the development of information technology, the wide-scale production of computers, the development of user-friendly software, and the educational applications that followed have all had profound effects on the way we learn and the way we teach (Heller, Ortos, & Crowley, 2000). This chapter explores the challenges and opportunities resulting from the use of technology as they pertain to health and health-care education by nurses and professional education for nurses. [3]

I. **HEALTH EDUCATION IN THE INFORMATION AGE**

The use of technology in education reflects what is happening on a much larger scale in our communities. Hence, it is useful to think of educational technology within the broader context of the environment in which we live and work.

We are in a period of history often referred to as the *Information Age*. Mitchel and McCullough (1995) describe the Information Age as a place in time when sweeping advances in computer and information technology have transformed the economic, social, and cultural life of society. If you think about the many ways in which technology has changed the world we live in, it is clear that computers have become more than tools to make life easier—they have become part of our culture.

The use of Information Age technology has had such a dramatic influence on health education that a new and rapidly expanding field of study, consumer informatics, has emerged. **Consumer informatics**, also referred to as **consumer health informatics**, is defined as a discipline that "analyses consumers' needs for information, studies and implements methods of making information accessible to consumers, and models and integrates consumer preferences into medical information systems" (Eysenbach, 2000, p. 1713). [2]

II. THE IMPACT OF TECHNOLOGY ON THE TEACHER AND THE LEARNER

Information Age technology has had a significant influence on educators and learners in all educational settings (Gross, 1999). Access to information bridges the gap between student and teacher. When information is widely available, the teacher is no longer the person who holds all of the answers or the individual who is solely responsible for imparting knowledge. Therefore, educators in the Information Age are becoming facilitators of learning rather than providers of information and are striving to create a collaborative atmosphere in their teaching and learning environments.

As information becomes more and more accessible, the need for memorization becomes less important than the ability to think critically. Hence, educators in the Information Age are helping individuals learn how to refine a problem, find the information they need, and critically evaluate the information they find. Healthcare education can and should follow a similar path. As educators, nurses must learn how and when to use technology and modify their educational approaches to be consistent with the needs of Information Age clients. Nurses must strive to be facilitators of learning and create learning environments in which clients are encouraged and supported to seek the information they need to achieve optimum health.[3]

STRATEGIES FOR USING TECHNOLOGY IN HEALTHCARE EDUCATION

The World Wide Web

The technology-based educational resource that is familiar to most people is the World Wide Web. One merely has to turn on a television and hear the commercials for health-related Websites or hear references to the Web on morning talk shows to appreciate its tremendous influence.

Having recognized the value of the World Wide Web, nurses and other healthcare educators are beginning to teach their clients how to use the Web to find the resources and health- care information they need to become educated healthcare consumers.

The Internet

The World Wide Web is merely a small component of a much larger computer network called the Internet. Although the Internet does not provide the eye-catching Web pages and the multimedia found on the World Wide Web, it does offer a wide range of services, many of which can be used to deliver health and healthcare education to clients.

III. ISSUES RELATED TO THE USE OF TECHNOLOGY

Despite the power of computer and Internet technology to enhance learning, the use of these technologies in healthcare education presents some unique challenges. Think for a moment about the many ways in which healthcare education differs from more traditional classroom education. The characteristics of the learners, the setting, and the access to hardware, software, and technological support are all likely to be different.

Whereas traditional classroom education is likely to take place in a structured setting, healthcare education takes place in a wide range of settings, many of which are unstructured. Students who are part of an educational system are likely to access the hardware, software, and technological support necessary for facilitating technology-based learning.

By comparison, access to resources and support varies considerably among healthcare consumers and in healthcare organizations. Students in a classroom also often share many common characteristics related to age and ability, whereas clients in healthcare education programs may cover a wide range of ages, abilities, and limitations. As educators, nurses must be aware of the special issues involved in the use of computer and Internet technology in healthcare education and be prepared to make accommodations as needed. [3]

Digital Divide and Digital Inclusion

One of the most widely publicized issues related to the use of computers and Internet technology is that of the **digital divide**, or the gap between those individuals who have access to information technology resources and those who do not. As a result of the digital divide, many healthcare consumers do not have the resources necessary to gain entry to computer- and Internet-based health education programs. Thus, although technology can increase access to healthcare education for some people, educators must be aware that large segments of the population will be denied access if attempts are not made to promote "**digital inclusion**."

The first step in promoting digital inclusion is recognizing those groups who are at risk for limited access. Health and healthcare education is important to senior citizens, and computer- and Internet-based technology holds much promise for this segment of the population. Therefore, it is important that the nurse be prepared to support computer-based learning among older clients.

The following interventions may be helpful in encouraging senior citizens to engage in computer-based learning activities:

1. *Reinforce principles of ergonomics* by making suggestions about equipment and posture that will minimize physical problems related to computer use.
2. *Identify resources* that will provide computer access and support in the senior citizen's home community.
3. *Motivate older adults* to use a computer by helping them to identify how the computer can meet their needs
4. Cre*ate a supportive and non-threatening environment* to teach older adults about using a computer for health education.

IV. PROFESSIONAL EDUCATION

From work-site training to higher education, technology makes professional education more accessible and meaningful for nurses. It is no longer necessary for nurses to quit working or to relocate to earn a higher degree. Technology has contributed to the growth of distance education programs at all levels in nursing. Likewise, technology makes it possible for nurses in the workplace to engage in various educational activities designed to keep their practice current, provide career mobility, and enhance professional development.

E-Learning

Technology has impacted workforce training that it has given birth to a new industry and a new set of buzzwords that define an Information Age approach to staff education. Professional development and training organizations have capitalized on the power of computer technology to provide businesses with learning solutions referred to as *e-learning*, an abbreviation for electronic learning. [3]

Distance Education

As a result of technological advances, distance education for nurses is flourishing in the twenty-first century (Potempa et al., 2001). The term *distance learning* means different things to different people. Online courses, correspondence courses, independent study, and videoconferencing are just a few of the techniques that can be used to deliver education to students studying at a distance.

Online courses provide learning activities and resources and facilitate teacher-learner and learner-learner interactions. Internet-based courses might work very well in areas such as parenting and diabetes education where there is an extended program of instruction and the need for group support.

SUMMARY

This chapter focused on Information Age technology and its use in healthcare education. Specifically, the chapter discussed ways in which nurse educators could use the World Wide Web and the Internet to enhance health and healthcare education for consumers and healthcare professionals. The impact of technology on teachers and learners was addressed and special considerations for older adults were identified. Trends in distance education for nurses were also explored. Information Age technology has the potential to transform health and healthcare education. This powerful tool must be used thoughtfully and carefully, however. Education is about learning, not about technology. Technology is merely an enhancement, a vehicle to deliver educational programs and to promote learning. The benefits of technology-based education are numerous, as are the challenges for educators and learners. As nurses, we have a responsibility to learn to use this new tool to promote health in our clients and professional growth and development in ourselves. The future for health education looks very bright. We can help shape it by continuing to think creatively about how to use technology in education and by participating in research about its effectiveness.

REVIEW QUESTIONS

1. What is the "Information Age" and how has it influenced education in general, healthcare education specifically, and healthcare consumers?

2. What Information Age skills do healthcare professionals and healthcare consumers require?

3. How can resources on the World Wide Web be used as a health information resource for healthcare consumers and healthcare professionals?

4. What are the various ways in which the Internet can be used to facilitate electronic communication between and among nurse educators and healthcare consumers? What are the advantages and disadvantages of each?

5. When using computer resources with clients, which segments of the population require special considerations due to limited access or special needs? What are those considerations and how can they be addressed?

6. What is e-learning and what advantages does it offer in providing training in healthcare settings?

7. How has technology influenced professional and continuing education options for nurses?

CHAPTER 13
INSTRUCTIONAL SETTINGS

Overview:

This chapter will examine the trends in health care affecting the delivery of instruction in various settings, classify instructional settings in which health teaching takes place, present a comparative analysis of the variables affecting educational efforts within different practice environments, and recommend teaching strategies best suited for specific settings in which teaching and learning take place.

Learning Outcomes

After completing this chapter, the student will be able to:

1. Recognize the trends in health care that are expanding opportunities and expectations of the nurse in the role of educator.
2. Classify the instructional setting in which the role of the nurse as an educator is played out.
3. Describe the factors that affect the nurse in the role of educator in each setting.
4. Select the preferred teaching strategies for each instructional setting.

INSTRUCTIONAL SETTINGS

Because health education is an integral component of nursing practice and has become an increasingly important responsibility of nurses in all practice environments, it is imperative to examine the factors influencing the teaching-learning process in various settings where clients - well or ill, are consumers of health care. The chief difference in the delivery of nursing care in acute care and long-term care facilities versus community-based environments is not only in the health status of the client but also in the length of time and resources available for educational activities. This chapter will examine the trends in health care affecting the delivery of instruction in various settings; classify instructional settings in which health teaching takes place; present a comparative analysis of the variables affecting educational efforts within different practice environments, and recommend teaching strategies best suited for specific settings in which teaching and learning take place.

I. EMERGING TRENDS IN HEALTH CARE

The major trends affecting the healthcare system come from healthcare economics coupled with advances in medical technology. As a result, patients are being discharged "quicker" and "sicker," with many of them receiving sophisticated treatment modalities outside the acute care environment. This has forced providers to cope with the challenge of delivering high-tech, complex care in less structured and at times less supportive community environments, with clients and their families having to assume increasingly more responsibility for the ongoing management of the medical regimen within their homes.

With the increased focus on prevention, promotion, and independence in self-care activities, today's newly emerging healthcare system mandates the education of consumers to a greater extent than ever before. Opportunities for client teaching have become increasingly more varied in terms of the types of clients encountered, their particular learning needs, and the settings in which health teaching occurs.

For health education to have a meaningful impact on the lives of others, nurse educators must have a sound understanding of the teaching-learning process to take advantage of the multitude of opportunities to educate consumers. They are also expected to be increasingly adept at identifying the type of content and instructional methodologies that most effectively and efficiently deliver the intended health messages. Additionally, nurses need to become knowledgeable about the Internet as a major source of information in the health education of clients (Desborough, 1999).

II. CLASSIFICATION OF INSTRUCTIONAL SETTINGS

A. Instructional Setting

An *instructional setting* is conceptualized based on the relationship health education has to the organization's primary function, agency, or institution within which it occurs. It is an entity whose fundamental mission is to provide health care, engage in health care activities, or be involved primarily in activities unrelated to health care. Based on this perspective, three types of settings for the education of clients have been identified:

B. Healthcare Setting

A *healthcare setting* is one in which the delivery of health care is the primary or sole function of the institution, organization, or agency. Hospitals, visiting nurse associations, public health departments, outpatient clinics, extended-care facilities, health maintenance organizations, physician offices, and nurse-managed centers are examples of organizations whose primary purpose is to deliver health care, for which health education is an integral aspect of the overall care delivered within these settings. Nurses function to provide direct patient care, and their role encompasses the teaching of clients as part of that care.

C. Healthcare-Related Setting

A *healthcare-related setting* is one in which healthcare-related services are offered as a complementary function of a quasi-health agency. Examples of this type of setting include the Philippine Heart Association, the Philippine Cancer Society, etc.

D. Non-Healthcare Setting

A *non-healthcare setting* is one in which health care is an incidental or supportive function of an organization. Examples of organizations classified as being this type of setting include businesses, industries, schools, and military and penal institutions.

The primary purpose of these organizations is to produce a manufactured product or offer a non–health-related service to the public. Industries, for example, are involved in health care only to the extent of providing health screenings and non-emergent health coverage to their employees through a health office within their place of employment, making available instruction in job-related health and safety issues to meet Occupational Safety and Health Administration (OSHA) regulations, or providing opportunities for health education through wellness programs to reduce absenteeism or improve employee morale.

Thus, an **instructional setting** is an environment in which health education takes place to provide individuals with the opportunity to engage in learning experiences for the purpose of improving their health or reducing their risk for illness

III. FACTORS RELATED TO INSTRUCTIONAL SETTING

These variables, which positively or negatively influence the success of teaching strategies and the outcomes of learning in any particular situation, are classified into three main categories: *organizational*, *environmental*, and *clientele factors*.

Organizational Factors

1. *What is the administrative perspective regarding health education?* The philosophy of the organization emanates from those who are in control of its operations. The attitude of the administration about the teaching of health information is of utmost importance to the success of educational endeavors. Administrative support influences the amount and types of resources available for education.

2. *How much time is allocated to the teaching of health information?* Regardless of the instructional setting, time is a valuable resource that exerts a major influence over the delivery of education to clients. The length of time a client remains in contact with the healthcare system for receipt of services is shrinking as a result of economic factors. Time for educational activities is often a scarce commodity within any organization but particularly in health-care agencies, where the amount of contact time with patients is being further limited by organizational responses to external healthcare reforms, resulting in fewer nurses for the same number or more clients.

3. *To what extent are resources available to carry out educational endeavors?* Sufficient financial support is required to ensure adequacy of nursing staff, the purchase of needed audiovisual materials and instructional equipment, time to develop content-specific materials, and the provision of space for teaching. Adequate resources make possible the implementation of efficient and effective educational interventions. Without the required resources, information fails to be consistently provided, and the specific needs of clients go unaddressed.

4. *Is the staff within the organization expert in the teaching role?* Although undergraduate nursing education may include principles of teaching and learning in patient education, a basic understanding is generally insufficient to prepare nurses to creatively integrate teaching into their demanding work schedules. In a healthcare environment, the informal reward system often recognizes physical care as more important than the teaching of self-care. Nurses frequently view patient care as a series of tasks rather than as an interactive process to support the development of new skills by the client.

5. *What is the level of support from physicians and other colleagues?* Although a growing number of nurse educators are quite capable of identifying clients' learning needs and providing for the education to meet those needs, in healthcare settings physician support is imperative in providing for that education. Within healthcare organizations, instituting innovative client education approaches is facilitated when the support of physicians and other professional colleagues is present (Shendell-Falik, 1990). Good communication and positive relationships among

colleagues are necessary to provide continuity of care, which includes patient education as one very important aspect of overall treatment.

Environmental Factors

1. *What external resources are available within the environment to support and promote the educational process?* The services of consultants and specialists from other healthcare disciplines, such as dieticians, occupational therapists, physicians, physical therapists, speech therapists, and social workers, must be available to complement the efforts by nurse educators in helping clients to acquire skills needed to attain or maintain optimal wellness

2. *What structural characteristics may stimulate or impede the development and use of educational programs?* Consideration must be given to location, travel time, space availability, costs, scheduling, and accessibility when designing a new program or continuing an existing one. The physical layout of a given area needs to be evaluated, with attention being paid to its adequacy for client privacy, low distraction potential, roominess, comfort, and ability to easily accommodate equipment related to the topics and skills being taught.

Clientele Factors

1. *What is the health status of the client?* The client who is well most likely has a low or moderate state of anxiety and is therefore likely to be receptive to teaching and learning. However, for the patient who is acutely or chronically ill, symptom distress such as fatigue, discomfort, and anxiety, along with the client and family's perceptions of the illness and support systems available, may adversely affect the person's ability to learn. For hospitalized individuals, the loss of personal control, lack of privacy, and social isolation can negatively affect their ability to actively participate in acquiring needed skills for self-care.

2. *What is the nature of the contact with the client over time?* Contact with the client is highly variable, depending on the situation. If the patient is hospitalized, the opportunity for frequent contact may be more

concentrated, over a week or just a few days or even hours

3. *What are the developmental levels, language skills, age, literacy levels, disabilities, and cultural beliefs of the client?* For settings that serve special populations or multilingual, low-literate, or culturally diverse groups, education methods and materials must be specifically designed to meet the needs of this clientele. The nurse educator must determine the homogeneity and heterogeneity of the populations in different settings when planning educational strategies.

4. *How self-directed is the client in seeking information?* A major goal of education is to gain the compliance of the learner in carrying out treatment regimens and self-care activities. Research on locus of control suggests that internally oriented individuals prefer to maintain self-control and are likely to be health-oriented, compliant with treatment regimens, and receptive to health teaching. Conversely, those with an external locus of control prefer to relinquish control to healthcare providers and present a challenge for the nurse educator in motivating them to attend educational sessions and actively participate in learning activities. This problem can become an even greater challenge to the health educator as the healthcare system demands more self-care responsibility from the client.

5. *How critical to the health and well-being of the learner is the educational content being presented?* If what is being taught is viewed as important information that can be used to help attain or maintain optimal health or reduce the likelihood of an emergency situation, then the clients' attention will be oriented to learning. If the learners do not see the relevance of the information to improving their lifestyle and health status, it is unlikely they will have much motivation for learning or participating in self-care.

6. *What resources are available to assist clients in achieving educational outcomes?* The clients' financial resources must be taken into account because they cannot be expected to follow a specific regimen of care if money to obtain the necessary equipment, medications, foods, or services prescribed is not available. Even healthy individuals who attend

programs for promotion of health and disease prevention may not have the financial resources to carry through with all suggested lifestyle changes. Psychosocial resources, such as the presence of supportive family members or significant others, are most beneficial to the learning experience because they can reinforce the teaching–learning process and provide assistance with self-care activities for those less able for whatever reason.

IV. <u>SHARING RESOURCES AMONG SETTINGS</u>

Professional nurses involved in client health education should use available opportunities to share resources among the three identified settings. Many already perform this service as printed or audiovisual materials are borrowed, rented, or purchased for small fees from area institutions, organizations, or agencies; nurse educators from healthcare or healthcare-related settings are contracted for or voluntarily provide health education programs to small and large groups in other healthcare, healthcare-related, or non-healthcare settings; and nurses from each category of setting collaborate on individual client situations or on major community health projects.

The nurses from each of these settings can establish a health education committee in their community to coordinate health education programming, ensure effective use of all resources, and reduce duplication of efforts. The members of this committee can develop standardized health education content, delineate roles and services for each of the instructional settings, and share resources to provide a well-planned, comprehensive community program of health education for a wide spectrum of clients

SUMMARY

Classification of instructional settings for client or patient education offers a method for analyzing the role of the nurse as educator and for selecting teaching strategies that best fit the organizational climate, the resources available, and the clientele served. Instructional settings are classified according to the purpose of the organization, institution, or agency that provides or sponsors health instruction. Healthcare settings exist for the primary purpose of providing direct patient care, with education occurring as an integral part of healthcare delivery services within the setting. Healthcare-related settings consist of voluntary agencies whose purposes are advocacy, research, and educating the general public as well as professionals regarding specific healthcare problems affecting society. Non-healthcare settings include institutions engaged in anything other than health care as their operational purpose, though they may choose to provide health education or health- care services as benefits to their membership or employees. The factors that affect instructional settings are directly related to the organization that provides the education, the environmental resources available, and the clientele who are serviced by the health education program. These factors need to be assessed prior to engaging in health education activities or selecting teaching strategies appropriate for the instructional setting. As always, the learning needs and characteristics of the learners are the major determinants in choosing the teaching strategies to be used in any setting. Teaching methods must be expanded to include multisensory, technologically advanced media to provide greater individualization and reach increasing numbers of clients.

CONTENT EVALUATION

The evaluation after the end of this chapter will be done through a take-home quiz, which the students must answer. Citations from other sources must be referenced by way of footnotes. Each paper will go through a plagiarism checker to ensure that none of the answers are copy-pasted. The output shall be submitted through e-mail and shall form part of the student's overall grade.

REVIEW QUESTIONS

1. What are the trends in health care expanding the opportunities and expectations of the nurse in the role of educator?
2. What are the three (3) classifications of instructional settings?
3. Give five (5) examples of organizations, institutions, or agencies identified as health- care settings
4. Give five (5) examples of organizations, institutions, or agencies identified as healthcare-related settings
5. Give five (5) examples of organizations, institutions, or agencies identified as non-healthcare settings
6. What is the concept upon which instructional settings are classified?

7. What are the three (3) major factors influencing instructional settings?
8. What are the preferred teaching strategies for each instructional setting?

CHAPTER 14
EVALUATION IN HEALTHCARE EDUCATION

Overview:

Evaluation is a process within a process, and it's an important part of the nursing, decision-making, and educational processes. Each of these steps concludes with an evaluation. Because these processes are cyclical, assessment acts as a vital link at the conclusion of one cycle, guiding the following cycle's direction. Each part of the assessment process is critical, but none of them are meaningful unless the evaluation results are used to guide future planning and implementation of educational interventions. [1]

Learning Objectives

The student will be able to do the following after finishing this chapter:

1. Distinguish between evaluation and assessment.
2. Determine the evaluation's goals.
3. Recognize the five different types of evaluations: process, content, outcome, impact, and program.
4. Compare and contrast the characteristics of various evaluation models.
5. Identify evaluation roadblocks.

IN HEALTHCARE EDUCATION, EVALUATION

The process of evaluation allows us to demonstrate that what we do as nurses and nurse educators adds value to the care we offer. The term "evaluation" refers to a systematic procedure for determining the worth or value of anything, in this case, teaching and learning. In today's healthcare environment, early consideration of evaluation is more important than ever. The consequences of learning are crucial in making important decisions about learners. Is it possible for the patient to return home? Is the nurse capable of providing competent care? If education is to be justified as a value-added activity, the educational process must be measurable and measurable outcomes must be measurable. Education must produce measurable results for both the student and the enterprise. [1], [2], [3], [4], [5], [6], [

I. ASSESSMENT VS. EVALUATION

While assessment and evaluation are closely connected and are sometimes used interchangeably, they are not interchangeable concepts. The goal of the assessment process is to collect, synthesize, evaluate, and apply data to choose a course of action. The goal of evaluation is to collect, synthesize, evaluate, and apply data to judge the success of a certain action. [3]

The main distinctions between the two phrases are in terms of chronology and intent. An education program, for example, begins with a needs assessment of the students. Assessment data could be referred to as "input" in the context of systems theory. Periodic review during the program allows the educator to see if the program and learners are progressing as expected. Following the completion of the program, evaluation determines whether and to what degree the identified needs were addressed. These evaluative data could be referred to as "intermediate output" and "output," respectively, in terms of systems theory.

Assessment and evaluation planning should ideally take place simultaneously. Use the same data gathering methods and instruments whenever possible. This method is particularly well suited to outcome and impact evaluations.

II. SELECTING THE EVALUATION FOCUS

The first and most important step in any evaluation preparation process is establishing the evaluation's focus. The evaluation's design, conduct, data analysis, and reporting of outcomes will all be guided by this objective. It is impossible to overstate the necessity of a clear, focused, and realistic evaluation emphasis. The usefulness and correctness of an evaluation's results are significantly influenced by how well the evaluation is first focused.

The audience, goal, questions, scope, and resources are the five essential components of an evaluation focus (Ruzicki, 1987). Ask yourself the following questions to figure out what these elements are:

1. Who is the evaluation being carried out for? Audience

2. What is the purpose of the evaluation? Purpose
3. What types of questions will be asked throughout the assessment? Questions
4. What is the evaluation's scope? Scope
5. What are the resources available for the evaluation? Resources

Audience

• The audience is made up of the people or groups for whom the evaluation is being carried out (Ruzicki, 1987). The primary audience, or the person or group who requested the evaluation, and the wider audience, or everyone who will use or profit from the evaluation results, are among these persons or groups. Patients, peers, your supervisor, the nursing director, the staff development director, the chief executive officer of your institution, or a gathering of community leaders could all be part of an evaluation's audience.

• You will provide comments to all members of the audience when you present the evaluation results. However, when focusing the evaluation, keep the primary audience in mind. Giving precedence to the person or group who requested the evaluation will make it easier to focus the evaluation, especially if the results will be used by various parties with different interests.

Purpose

• The evaluation's objective is to provide an answer to the question, "Why is the evaluation being conducted?" An evaluation may be used to determine whether or not to continue a particular educational program or to assess the effectiveness of the teaching process. Use feedback from that group to explain the purpose if a certain individual or group has a primary interest in the evaluation's conclusions.

Questions

• The questions to be answered in the evaluation are directly related to the evaluation's aim, are specific, and are measurable. "How satisfied are patients with the cardiac discharge teaching program?" and "How frequently do staff nurses use the diabetes teaching reference materials?" are two examples of queries.

• If the evaluation is to achieve its goal, it is critical to ask the proper questions.

Scope

• An evaluation's scope might be thought of as an answer to the question, "How much will be evaluated?" "Will there be evaluations of how many areas of education?", "Will there be evaluations of how many persons or representative groups?", and "Will there be evaluations of how long?"

• Will the evaluation, for example, focus on one class or an entire program; on one patient's learning experience or all patients being taught a certain skill?

Resources

• Time, expertise, employees, resources, equipment, and facilities are all needed to conduct an evaluation. Focusing any evaluation requires a realistic assessment of what resources are accessible and available in relation to what resources are necessary.

• Don't forget to include in the time and skill required to collect, analyze, and interpret data, as well as the time and experience required to compile the assessment outcomes report.

Based on one or more of the five components stated above, evaluation can be categorized into several sorts or categories. Process, content, outcome, impact, and program evaluation are the most common forms of assessment identified.

EVALUATION MODELS

For conceiving or defining educational evaluation into distinct categories or levels, Abruzzese (1978) established the Roberta Straessle Abruzzese (RSA) Evaluation Model. The RSA Model is effective for understanding different sorts of evaluations from the perspectives of both staff development and patient education.

Based on the aim and related questions, scope, and resource components of evaluation focus, the RSA Model graphically places five fundamental forms of assessment in relation to one another. Process, content, outcome, impact, and program are the five categories of evaluation. The first four forms are described by Abruzzese as levels of evaluation, ranging from simple (process evaluation) to complicated (system evaluation) (impact evaluation). All four levels are included and summarized in a whole program evaluation.

1. Formative (process) evaluation

• The goal of process or formative evaluation is to make changes to an educational activity as soon as possible, whether those changes be in staff, resources, facilities, learning objectives, or even one's own attitude.

• The scope of process assessment is often limited in breadth and time span to a single learning experience, such as a class or workshop, but it is sufficiently detailed to encompass as many components of that learning experience as feasible while they are occurring. Within the purview of process evaluation, learner behavior, teacher conduct, learner-teacher interaction, learner response to teaching materials and methods, and environmental features are all parts of the learning experience.

2. Content Assessment

• The goal of content evaluation is to see if students have learned the knowledge or abilities that were taught during the learning process.

• According to Abruzzese (1978), content evaluation occurs immediately following the learning experience in order to answer the guiding question, "To what extent did the learners learn what was imparted?" or "To what extent did students fulfill their goals?" Content evaluation can include things like asking a patient to do a follow-up demonstration or having attendees take a cognitive test at the end of a one-day seminar.

• In the RSA Model, content evaluation is shown as the level "in between" process and outcome assessment levels. To put it another way, content evaluation focuses on how the teaching-learning process influenced immediate, short-term outcomes.

3. Evaluation of the final result (summative)

• The goal of outcome evaluation is to figure out what the impacts or outcomes of your teaching efforts are. Because it aims to "sum" what happened as a result of schooling, outcome evaluation is also known as summative evaluation.

• Outcome evaluation occurs after teaching or after a program has been finished, just as process evaluation occurs concurrently with the teaching-learning activity. The change that occurs as a result of teaching and learning is measured through outcome evaluation.

• Abruzzese (1978) distinguishes outcome evaluation from content evaluation by emphasizing the latter's focus on long-term change that "remains after the learning experience" (p. 243). Institution of a new procedure, habitual usage of a new skill or behavior, or incorporation of a new value or attitude are all examples of changes.

• The scope of result evaluation is influenced by the changes being measured, which are in turn influenced by the educational activity's aims. As previously said, outcome evaluation considers a longer period of time than content evaluation. While content evaluation may involve testing a patient's proficiency with a skill in the home environment after discharge, outcome evaluation should include measuring a patient's competency with a skill in the home setting after discharge.

4. Impact Assessment

• The goal of impact evaluation is to figure out how education affects the institution or the community. To put it another way, the goal of impact evaluation is to gather data that will aid in determining whether or not continuing an educational activity is worthwhile.

• Impact evaluations have a broader, more complicated, and typically longer scope than process, content, or outcome evaluations. Whereas outcome evaluation would look at whether a given teaching method led to the achievement of specific results, impact evaluation would look at the impact or value of those outcomes. To put it another way, outcome evaluation is concerned with a course objective, whereas impact evaluation is concerned with a course goal.

• Take, for instance, a class on how to use body mechanics. The end goal is for staff workers to display good body mechanics while delivering patient care. The goal is to reduce back injuries among direct-care providers at the hospital. Although the distinction between outcome and impact evaluations may appear minor, it is critical to the proper design and execution of an impact evaluation.

5. Evaluation of the Program

• The goal of program assessment can be summarized as "planned and conducted to aid an audience in judging and improving the value of some product" (Johnson & Olesinski, 1995, p. 53). In this situation, the "object" is an educational program.

• The goal of whole program evaluation, as defined by the RSA Model (Abruzzese, 1978), is to assess the extent to which all activities for an entire department or program over a specific period of time match or surpass the initial goals.

• Program evaluation has a broad scope, concentrating on overall goals rather than individual targets. The scope of program assessment, according to Abruzzese (1978), includes all areas of educational activity (e.g., process, content, outcome, and impact) with input from all participants (e.g., learners, teachers, institutional representatives, community representatives). Depending on the time frame chosen for fulfilling the goals to be reviewed, the data collection period can range from a few months to one or more years.

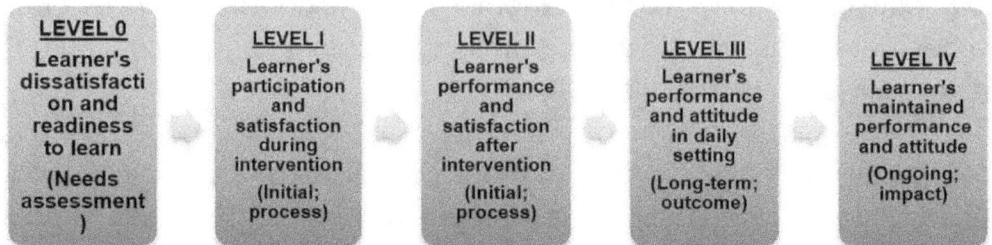

Figure 1. **Five Levels of Learner Evaluation** SOURCE: Based on S. H. Rankin & K. D. Stallings (2001). *Patient Education: Principles and Practices*, 4th ed. Philadelphia: Lippincott.

I. DESIGNING THE EVALUATION

An evaluation's design must be compatible with the evaluation's objective, questions, and scope, as well as feasible given available resources. Structure, methodology, and instruments are at least three interrelated components of evaluation design.

A. Structure Design

• "How rigorous should the evaluation be?" is a crucial issue to consider while designing an evaluation. The obvious response is that all evaluations should be rigorous in some way. To put it another way, all evaluations should be systematic, well-planned, and well-structured before they are carried out.

Research vs. Evaluation

• The terms "evaluation" and "research" are not interchangeable or mutually exclusive. The degree to which they are substantially different or indistinguishable from one another is determined by the type of evaluation and research being evaluated.

• According to Ruzicki (1987), there is a differentiation between the two: While both research and evaluation entail the collecting of objective, methodical data, evaluation is done to make decisions in a specific situation. Research is created in such a way that it can be generalized and duplicated in many circumstances.

B. Evaluation Techniques

• Determining the evaluation design structure is based on the evaluation emphasis. In turn, the design structure serves as the foundation for defining evaluation methodologies. The measures taken to carry out the evaluation in accordance with the design structure are referred to as evaluation procedures.

• All assessment approaches deal with data and data collection in some way. The answers to the following questions will help you choose the most appropriate and viable methods for performing a specific evaluation in a specific location and for a specific purpose:

a) What kinds of information will be gathered?

b) From whom or what will information be gathered?

c) How will data be gathered, when will it be collected, and where will it be collected?

d) Who will collect the data?

What Kinds of Information Should Be Gathered?

• Collecting data on people, the educational program or activity, and the setting in which the educational activity takes place are all part of the evaluation of healthcare education.

• Data regarding the people, the program, and the environment is required for process, result, impact, and program assessments. Although this limitation is unnecessary, content evaluations may be confined to data about the persons and the program.

• Data collected about humans can be classed as physical, cognitive, affective, or psychomotor in nature.

• Program features such as cost, length, number of educators necessary, amount and type of materials required, teaching-learning methods employed, and so on are among the data collected regarding educational activities or programs.

• Environmental parameters such as temperature, lighting, location, layout, space, and noise level are among the data collected about the environment in which a program or activity is undertaken.

Collecting Data from Whom or What

• Data can be obtained directly from the people whose behavior or knowledge is being assessed, through surrogates or representations, or from existing documentation or databases.

• Plan to obtain at least some data directly from individuals being evaluated wherever possible. When evaluating a process, data should be collected from all learners and educators who are involved in the educational activity. All learners' data should be included in content and outcome evaluations.

How, When, and Where Should Data Be Collected?

• Data can be acquired in a variety of ways, including:

a) Observatio
b) Interview
d) A questionnaire or a written test
d) Checking the records

a) Examination of existing databases on a secondary level

Instruments of Evaluation (C)

• First and foremost, the instrument must accurately measure the performance being evaluated as it has been operationally specified for the evaluation.

• Second, an appropriate instrument should have documented evidence of its reliability and validity with persons who are as similar to the people you will be collecting data as possible.

Evaluation Obstacles

There are three basic categories of obstacles to performing an evaluation:

1. An unclear, undeclared, or ill-defined evaluation focus is the most common cause of lack of clarity. It's tough to perform any action if the performer doesn't understand why they're doing it.

2. Inadequate understanding on how to perform an evaluation or insufficient or inaccessible resources to conduct the evaluation are the most common causes of inability to conduct an evaluation. The primary audience is frequently responsible for clarifying the evaluation purpose, questions, and scope. However, both the primary audience and the individuals doing the review are responsible for resource clarification.

3. Fear of being punished or losing one's self-esteem. Evaluation can be interpreted as a verdict on one's personal value. Individuals who are being evaluated may be concerned that anything less than faultless performance will result in punishment, or that their mistakes would be interpreted as proof that they are unworthy or inadequate as human beings. One of the most significant obstacles to performing an examination is fear. To overcome assessment hurdles, they must first be identified and understood, and then the evaluation must be structured and done in such a way that as many of the identified barriers as possible are minimized or eliminated.

II. **CONDUCTING THE EVALUATION**

To conduct an evaluation means to implement the evaluation design by using the instruments chosen or developed according to the methods selected. How smoothly an evaluation is implemented depends primarily on how carefully and thoroughly the evaluation was planned.

Three methods to minimize the effects of unexpected events that occur when carrying out an evaluation are to: (1) conduct a pilot test first, (2) include "extra" time, and (3) keep a sense of humor.

Conducting a pilot test of the evaluation entails trying out the data collection methods, instruments, and plan for data analysis with a few individuals who are the same as or very similar to those who will be included in the full evaluation. A pilot test must be conducted if any newly developed instruments are planned for the evaluation, to assess reliability, validity, interpretability, and feasibility of those new instruments.

Including "extra" time during the conduct of an evaluation means leaving room for the unexpected delays that almost invariably occur during evaluation planning, data collection, and translation of evaluation results into reports that will be meaningful and usable by the primary audience.

Because those delays not only will occur but also are likely to occur at inconvenient times during the evaluation, **keeping a sense of humor** is vitally important. An evaluator with a sense of humor is more likely to maintain a realistic perspective in reporting results that include negative findings, too. An audience with a vested interest in positive evaluation results may blame the evaluator if results are lower than expected.

III. <u>ANALYZING AND INTERPRETING DATA COLLECTED</u>

The purposes for conducting data analysis are (1) to organize data to provide meaningful information and (2) to provide answers to evaluation questions.

Data and **information** are not synonymous terms. That is, a mass of numbers or a mass of comments does not become information until it has been organized into coherent tables, graphs, or categories that are relevant to the purpose for conducting the evaluation.

Analysis of data should be consistent with the type of data collected. In other words, all data analysis must be rigorous, but not all data analysis need include use of inferential statistics. For example, qualitative data, such as verbal comments obtained during interviews and written comments obtained from open-ended questionnaires, are summarized or "themed" into categories of similar comments. Each category or theme is qualitatively described by directly quoting one or more comments that are typical of that category. These categories then may be quantitatively described using descriptive statistics such as total counts and percentages.

IV. REPORTING EVALUATION RESULTS

Results of an evaluation must be reported if the evaluation is to be of any use. Following a few guidelines when planning an evaluation will significantly increase the likelihood that results of the evaluation will be reported to the appropriate individuals or groups, in a timely manner, and in usable form:

a) **Be Audience Focused.** The purpose for conducting an evaluation is to provide information for decision-making by the primary audience. The report of evaluation results must, therefore, be consistent with that purpose. One rule of thumb to use: Always begin an evaluation report with an executive summary that is no longer than one page. No matter who the audience members are, their time is important to them. A second important guideline is to present evaluation results in a format and language that the audience can use and understand without additional interpretation. Third, make every effort to present results in person as well as in writing. Finally, include specific recommendations or suggestions for how evaluation results might be used.

b) **Stick to the Evaluation Purpose.** Keep the main body of an evaluation report focused on information that fulfills the purpose for conducting the evaluation. Provide answers to the questions asked. Include the main aspects of how the evaluation was conducted, but avoid a diary-like chronology of the activities of the evaluators.

c) **Stick to the Data.** Maintain consistency with actual data when reporting and interpreting findings. Keep in mind that a question not asked cannot be answered and that data not collected cannot be interpreted. If you did not measure or observe a teacher's performance, for example, do not draw conclusions about the adequacy of that performance. Similarly, if the only measures of patient performance were those conducted in the hospital, do not interpret successful inpatient performance as successful performance by the patient at home or at work.

A discussion of any limitations of the evaluation is an important part of the evaluation report. For example, if several patients were unable to complete a questionnaire because they could not understand it or because they were too fatigued, say so. Discussion of limitations also will provide useful information for what not to do the next time a similar evaluation is conducted.

SUMMARY

The process of evaluation in healthcare education involves gathering, summarizing, interpreting, and using data to determine the extent to which an educational activity is efficient, effective, and useful for those who participate in that activity as learners, teachers, or sponsors. Five types of evaluation were discussed in this chapter: process, content, outcome, impact, and program evaluations. Each of these types focuses on a specific purpose, scope, and questions to be asked of an educational activity or program to meet the needs of those who ask for the evaluation or who can benefit from its results. Each type of evaluation also requires some level of available resources for the evaluation to be conducted. A number of guidelines, rules of thumb, and suggestions have been included in this chapter's discussion of how a nurse educator might go about selecting the most appropriate model, design, methods, and instruments for a particular type of evaluation.

REVIEW QUESTIONS

1. How does the process of evaluation differ from the process of assessment?
2. What is the first and most crucial step in planning any evaluation?
3. What are the five (5) basic components included in determining the focus of an evaluation?
4. What are the five (5) basic types (levels) of evaluation in order from simple to complex identified in Abruzzese's RSA Evaluation Model?
5. How does *formative evaluation* differ from *summative evaluation* and what is another name for each of these two types of evaluation?
6. What is the purpose of each type (level) of evaluation as described by

Abruzzese in her RSA Evaluation Model?
7. What data collection methods can be used in conducting an evaluation of educational interventions?
8. What are the three (3) major barriers to conducting an evaluation?
9. When and why should a pilot test be conducted prior to implementing a full evaluation?
10. What are the three (3) guidelines to follow in reporting the results of an evaluation?

NOTES

Chapter 1
1. DeSantis, L. A., & Lipson, J. G. (2007). Brief history of inclusion of content on culture in nursing education. *Journal of Transcultural Nursing, 18*(1_suppl), 7S-9S. From <https://scholar.google.com/scholar?hl=en&as_sdt=0%2C5&q=a
2. Noble, M. A., Redmond, G. M., Williams, J. K., & Langley, C. (1996). Education for the nurse tomorrow: a community-focused curriculum. *N & Hc: Perspectives on Community, 17*(2), 66-72. From <https://scholar.google.com/scholar?hl=en&as_sdt=0%2C5&q=curriculum+common>

   Cole, A. L., & Knowles, J. G. (1993). Teacher development partnership research: A focus on methods and issues. *American educational research journal, 30*(3), 473-495. From <https://scholar.google.com/scholar?hl=en&as_sdt=0%2C5&q=Knowles%2C+1989+t>
4. Glanville, I., Schirm, V., & Wineman, N. M. (2000). Using evidence-based practice for managing clinical outcomes in advanced practice nursing. *Journal of Nursing Care Quality, 15*(1), 1-11. From <https://scholar.google.com/scholar?hl=en&as_sdt=0%2C5&q=process+infor>

Chapter 2
1. Nelson, M. J. (2003). Ethical, legal, and economic foundations of the educational process. *Nurse as educator: Principles of teaching and learning for nursing practice*, 21-41. From <https://scholar.google.com/scholar?hl=en&as_sdt=0%2C5&q=%28Lesnick+and+Andn>
2. Brent, N. J. (2001). *Nurses and the Law.* 2nd ed. Philadelphia: Saunders.
3. Abruzzese, R. S. (1992). *Nursing Staff Development: Strategies for Success.* St. Louis: Mosby.
4. Goldenberg, D., Andrusyszyn, M. A., & Iwasiw, C. (2005). The effect of classroom simulation on nursing students' self-efficacy related to health teaching. *Journal of Nursing Education, 44*(7), 310-314. From <https://scholar.google.com/scholar?hl=en&as_sdt=0%2C5&q=Boyd+et+al.%
5. Rothenberg, M. L., Abbruzzese, J. L., Moore, M., Portenoy, R. K., Robertson, J. M., & Wanebo, H. J. (1996). A rationale for expanding the endpoints for clinical trials in advanced pancreatic carcinoma. *Cancer: Interdisciplinary International Journal of the American Cancer Society, 78*(S3), 627-632. From

<https://scholar.google.com/scholar?hl=en&as_sdt=0%2C5&q=Abruzzese%2C+1992>

Chapter 3

1. Bigge, M. L., & Shermis, S. S. (1992). How does Bruner's cognitive psychology treat learning and teaching. *Learning theories for teachers.(5th ed.) New York: HarperCollins*, 123-146.*From* <https://scholar.google.com/scholar?hl=en&as_sdt=0%2C5&q=+%28Bigge+%26+Sher>
2. Hilgard, E. R., & Bower, G. H. (1966). Theories of learning. *From* <https://scholar.google.com/scholar?hl=en&as_sdt=0%2C5&q=Hilgard+%26+Bowern>
3. Levis, D. J., Klein, S. B., & Mowrer, R. R. (1989). The case for a return to a two-factor theory of avoidance: The failure of non-fear interpretations*From* <https://scholar.google.com/scholar?hl=en&as_sdt=0%2C5&q=Klein+%26+Mowrer%>
4. Levis, D. J., Klein, S. B., & Mowrer, R. R. (1989). The case for a return to a two-factor theory of avoidance: The failure of non-fear interpretations.*From* <https://scholar.google.com/scholar?hl=en&as_sdt=0%2C5&q=Klein+%26+Mowrer%n>
5. Brien, R., & Eastmond, N. (1994). *Cognitive science and instruction*. Educational Technology *From* <https://scholar.google.com/scholar?hl=en&as_sdt=0%2C5&q=Brien+%26+Eastmon>
6. Tatman, A. W., & Gilgen, A. R. (1999). Authorities and research emphasized in the Annual Review of Psychology, 1975–1998. *Psychological reports*, 85(1), 89-100.*From* <https://scholar.google.com/scholar?hl=en&as_sdt=0%2C5&q=Tatman+%26+Gilgen>

Chapter 4

1. McCoy, L. P., & Haggard, C. S. (1989). Determinants of Computer Use by Teachers. *From<https://scholar.google.com/scholar?hl=en&as_sdt=0%2C5&q=+determinants+o>*
2. Beers, G. W. (2005). The effect of teaching method on objective test scores: Problem-based learning versus lecture. *Journal of Nursing Education*, 44(7), 305-309. *From*

<https://scholar.google.com/scholar?hl=en&as_sdt=0%2C5&q=Musinski%2C+1999+a>
3. Corbett, C. F. (2003). A randomized pilot study of improving foot care in home health patients with diabetes. *The Diabetes Educator, 29*(2), 273-282. From <https://scholar.google.com/scholar?hl=en&as_sdt=0%2C5&q=patient+outcon>
4. Bakas, T., Farran, C. J., Austin, J. K., Given, B. A., Johnson, E. A., & Williams, L. S. (2009). Content validity and satisfaction with a stroke caregiver intervention program. *Journal of Nursing Scholarship, 41*(4), 368-375. From <https://scholar.google.com/scholar?hl=en&as_sdt=0%2C5&q=satisfaction+%28Bak>
5. Saunders, G. H., Field, D. L., & Haggard, M. P. (1992). A clinical test battery for obscure auditory dysfunction (OAD): development, selection and use of tests. *British journal of audiology, 26*(1), 33-42. From <https://scholar.google.com/scholar?hl=en&as_sdt=0%2C5&q=attending+to+the+thr>
6. Bonham, L. A. (1988). Learning style instruments: Let the buyer beware. *Lifelong Learning, 11*(6), 14–17.
7. Friedman, P. & Alley, R. (1984). Learning/teaching styles: Applying the principles. *Theory into Prac- tice, 23*(1), 77–81.
8. Kitchie S. (2012). Determinants of Learning. Jones & Bartlett Learning, LLC
9. https://nursekey.com/determinants-of-learning/

Chapter 5

1. Havighurst, R. J. (1976). Education through the adult life span. *Educational Gerontology, 1*(1), 41-51. From <https://scholar.google.com/scholar?hl=en&as_sdt=0%2C5&q=Havighurst+%_>
2. Hussey, C. G., & Hirsh, A. M. (1983). Health education for children. *Topics in clinical nursing, 5*(1), 22-28. From <https://scholar.google.com/scholar?hl=en&as_sdt=0%2C5&q=%28Hussey+%>
3. Milligan, F. (1997). In defence of andragogy. Part 2: an educational process consistent with modern nursing's aims. *Nurse Education Today, 17*(6), 487-493. From <https://scholar.google.com/scholar?hl=en&as_sdt=0%2C5&q=%28Milligan%>

4. Reeber, B. J. (1992). Evaluating the effects of a family education intervention. *Rehabilitation Nursing, 17*(6), 332-336.From <https://scholar.google.com/scholar?hl=en&as_sdt=0%2C5&q=variables+infl>
5. Giloth, B. E. (1990). Promoting patient involvement: educational, organizational, and environmental strategies. *Patient education and counseling, 15*(1), 29-38. From <https://scholar.google.com/scholar?hl=en&as_sdt=0%2C5&q=Family+care-+>
6. Hartmann, R. A., & Kochar, M. S. (1994). The provision of patient and family education. *Patient education and counseling, 24*(2), 101-108.From <https://scholar.google.com/scholar?hl=en&as_sdt=0%2C5&q=healthcare+n>

Chapter 6

1. Themes, U. (2016, September 9). *Compliance, motivation, and health behaviors of the learner.* Nurse Key. https://nursekey.com/compliance-motivation-and-health-behaviors-of-the-learner/
   From <https://www.citefast.com/?s=APA7>
2. Nurse as Educator: Principles of Teaching and Learning for https://ebin.pub/nurse-as-educator-principles-of-teaching-and-learning-for-nursing-practice-5nbsped-2017030094-9781284127201.html
3. Let's examine... Health Literacy. http://choosehealth.utah.gov/healthcare/continuing-education/diabetes-webinar-series/archives/presentations-2013/January_healthliteracy.pdf
4. compliance and motivation and models of health educationx https://www.coursehero.com/file/61387126/compliance-and-motivation-and-models-of-health-educationpptx/
5. Nurse as Educator: Principles of Teaching and Learning for https://ebin.pub/nurse-as-educator-principles-of-teaching-and-learning-for-nursing-practice-5nbsped-2017030094-9781284127201.html
6. Richards E. (2012). Motivation, Compliance, and Health Behaviors of the Learner. Jones & Bartlett Learning, LLC
7. https://nursekey.com/compliance-motivation-and-health-behaviors-of-the-learner/
8. Ajzen, I. & Fishbein, M. (1980). Understanding Attitudes and Predicting Social Behavior. Englewood Cliffs, NJ: Prentice-Hall.
3. Atkinson, J. W. (1964). An Introduction to Motivation. Princeton, NJ: Van Nostrand.
4. Bandura, A. (1977). Self-efficacy: Toward a unifying theory of behavioral change. Psychological Review, 84(2), 191–215.

Chapter 7

1. Bastable S and Sopczyk D. (2012). Gender, Socioeconomic, and Cultural Attributes of the Learner
https://nursekey.com/gender-socioeconomic-and-cultural-attributes-of-the-learner/
2. Andrews, M. M. & Boyle, J. S. (1995). Transcultural nursing care. In Transcultural Concepts in Nursing Care, 2nd ed. Philadelphia: Lippincott.
3. Babcock, D. E. & Miller, M. A. (1994). Client Education: Theory and Practice. St. Louis: Mosby–Year Book.
4. Nurse as educator: principles of teaching and learning for nursing practice / [edited by] Susan B. Bastable. 3rd ed.Sudbury, Mass: Jones and Bartlett, c2008

Chapter 8

1. Boss, B. J. (1986). The neuroanatomical and neurophysiological basis for learning. *Journal of Neuroscience Nursing, 18*(5), 256–264.
2. Boyd, M. D., Gleit, C. J., Graham, B. A., & Whitman, N. I. (1998). *Health Teaching in Nursing Practice*, 3rd ed. Stamford, CT: Appleton & Lange.
3. https://nursekey.com/behavioral-objectives/

Chapter 9

1. Arends, R. I. (1994). *Learning to Teach*, 3rd ed. New York: McGraw-Hill.Babcock, D. E. & Miller, M. A. (1994). *Client Education: Theory and Practice*. St. Louis: Mosby–Year Book.
2. Baldwin, D., Hill, P., & Hanson, G. (1991). Performance of psychomotor skills: A comparison of two teaching strategies. *Journal of Nursing Education, 30*(8), 367–370
3. Andrusyszyn, M. A. (1989). Clinical evaluation of the affective domain. *Nurse Education Today, 9*(2), 75–81.Arends, R. I. (1994). *Learning to Teach*, 3rd ed. New York: McGraw-Hill.
4. https://nursekey.com/behavioral-objectives/

Chapter 10

1. Babcock, D. E. & Miller, M. A. (1994). *Client Education: Theory and Practice*. St. Louis: Mosby–Year Book.
2. Haggard, A. (1989). *Handbook of Patient Education*. Rockville, MD: Aspen.
3. https://nursekey.com/instructional-methods-and-settings/

Chapter 11

1. compliance and motivation and models of health educationx …. https://www.coursehero.com/file/61387126/compliance-and-motivation-and-models-of-health-educationpptx/
2. instructional material 7bx - Instructional Materials 11th …. https://www.coursehero.com/file/61387316/instructional-material-7bpptx/
3. Principles of learning& Education NUR 315. http://fac.ksu.edu.sa/sites/default/files/315_nur_contents.pdf
4. Instructional Materials | Nurse Key. https://nursekey.com/instructional-materials/
5. TCT 201: INSTRUCTIONAL TECHNOLOGY Topic: Instructional Media. https://profiles.uonbi.ac.ke/peterkyalo/files/lecture_7a_-_instructional_media.pdf
6. Learning - Term Paper. https://www.termpaperwarehouse.com/essay-on/Learning/135011
7. Babcock, D. E. & Miller, M. A. (1994). *Client Education: Theory and Practice*. St. Louis: Mosby–Year Book.
8. Kaihoi, B. H. (1987). Implementing use of learning resources in our technological age. Chapter 7 in C. E. Smith, *Patient Education: Nurses in Partnership with Other Health Professionals*. Philadelphia: Saunders.
9. https://nursekey.com/instructional-materials/

Chapter 12

1. Technology in Education. https://www.ifeet.org/files/TBL-7-October-2020---Technology-in-Education.pdf
2. Technology in Education | Nurse Key. https://nursekey.com/technology-in-education/
3. Technology in Education. https://www.ifeet.org/files/TBL-7-October-2020---Technology-in-Education.pdf
4. American Association of Colleges of Nursing Task Force on Distance Technology and Nursing Education. (1999). *White Paper: Distance Technology in Nursing Education*. Washington, DC: American Association of Colleges of Nursing.
5. Association of Colleges & Research Libraries. (2000). *Information Literacy Competency Standards for Higher Education*. Retrieved from the World Wide Web, April 2001, at *www.ala.org/acrl/ilintro.html*.

6. Bliss, J., Allibone, C., Bontempo, B., Flynn, T., & Valvano, N. (1998). Creating a Web site for online social support: Melanocyte. *Computers in Nursing, 16*(4), 203–207.
7. What does research tell us about technology and higher learning? *Change, 27*, 20–27. Retrieved from the World Wide Web, April 2001, at http://www.learner.org/edtech/rscheval/rightquestion.html.
9. https://nursekey.com/technology-in-education/

Chapter 13
1. Boyd M. D., Gleit, C. J., Graham, B. A., & Whitman, N. I. (1998). *Health Teaching in Nursing Practice: A Professional Model*, 3rd ed. Stamford, CT: Apple- ton & Lange.
2. Breckon, D. J., Harvey, R. J., & Lancaster, R. B. (1985). *Community Health Education: Settings, Roles and Skills*. Rockville, MD: Aspen.
3. Davidhizar, R., Bechtel, G., & Dowd, S. B. (1998). Patient education: A mandate for health care in the 21st century. *Journal of Nuclear Medicine Technology, 26*(4), 235

CHAPTER 14
1. Evaluation in Healthcare Education. http://www.ifeet.org/files/TBL-2-May-8,-2018-Evaluation-in-Health-Care-Education.pdf
2. CHAPTER 15 Evaluation in Healthcare https://www.coursehero.com/file/97846508/CHAPTER-15docx/
3. Abruzzese, R.S. (1978). Evaluation in nursing staff development. In *Nursing Staff Development: Strategies for Success*. St. Louis: Mosby–Year Book.
4. Appling, S. E., Naumann, P. L., & Berk, R. A. (2001). Using a faculty evaluation triad to achieve evidence-based teaching. *Nursing and Health Care Perspectives, 22*(5), 247–251. http://www.ifeet.org/files/TBL-2-May-8,-2018-Evaluation-in-Health-Care-Education.pdf

www.ingramcontent.com/pod-product-compliance
Lightning Source LLC
Chambersburg PA
CBHW080959170526
45158CB00010B/2844